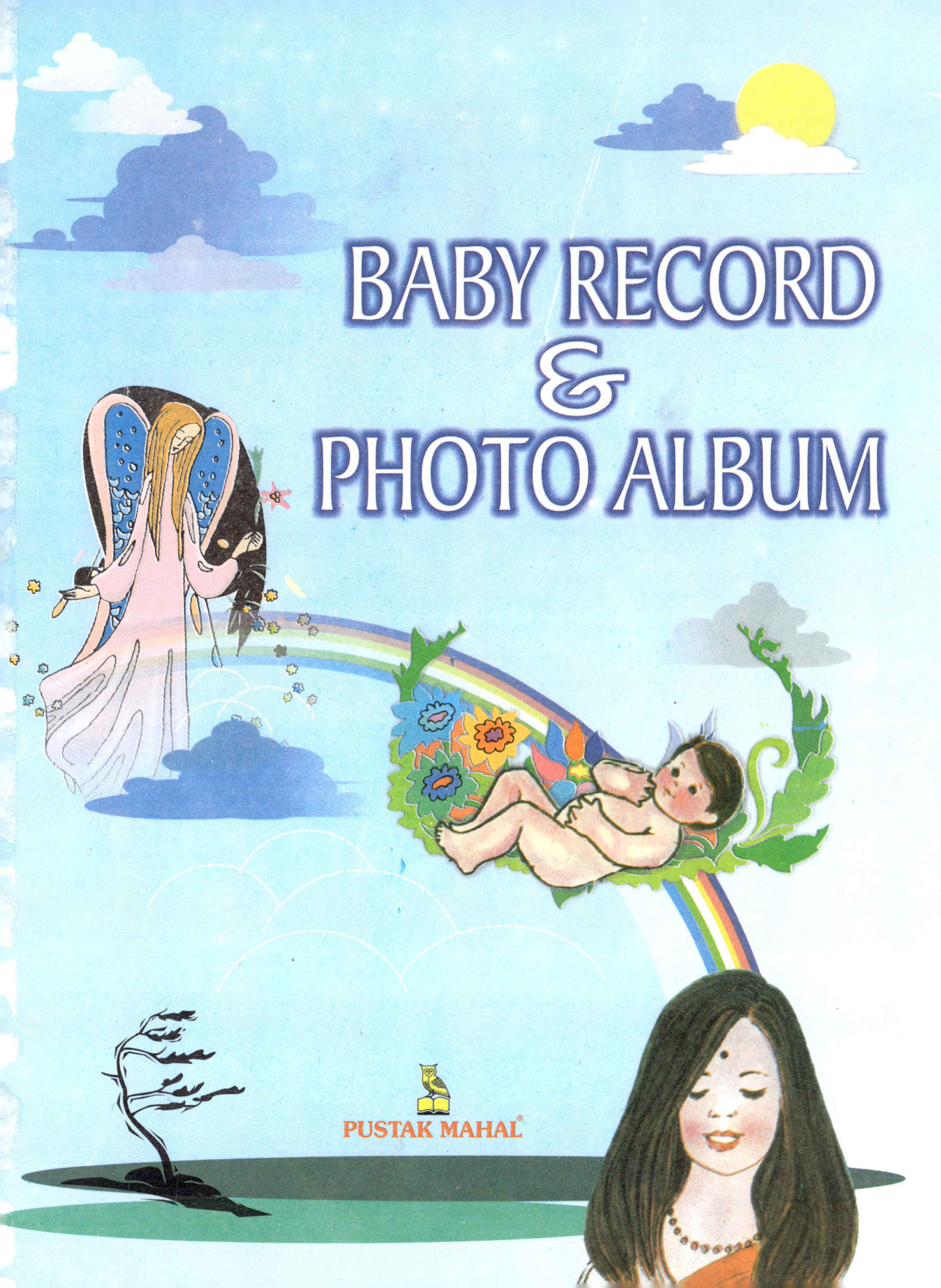
BABY RECORD
&
PHOTO ALBUM
PUSTAK MAHAL®

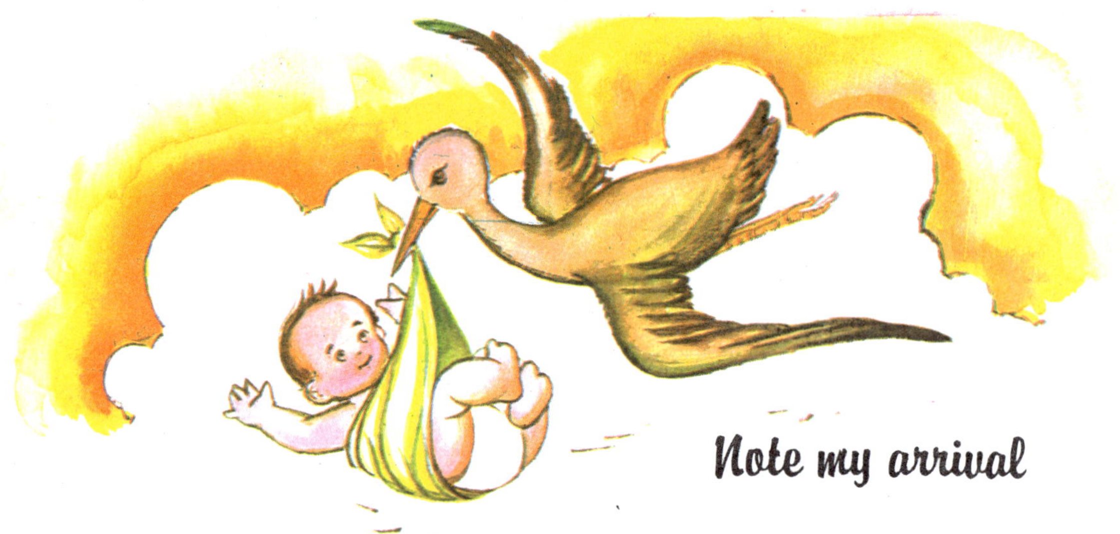

Note my arrival

Date of Birth ______________________ Time of Birth ____________________

Place __________________ Place among Brothers/Sisters ________________

Name of Doctor/Nurse/Midwife ____

Mother's ____________________________ Age __________________________

Father's ____________________________ Age __________________________

Photograph

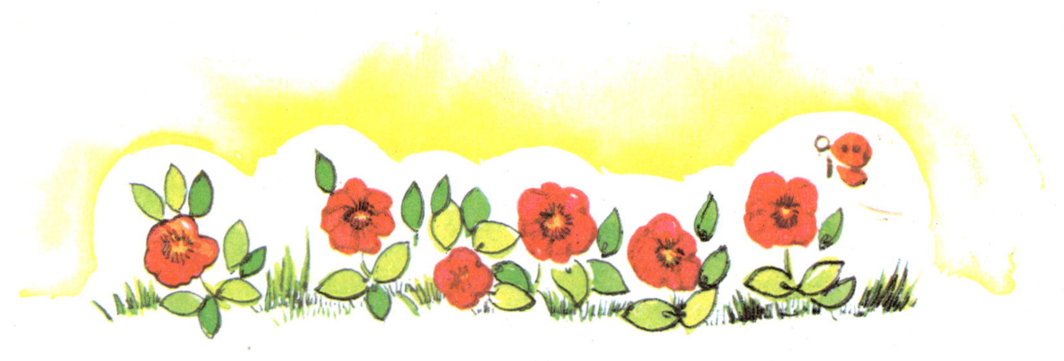

Particulars at birth

Length ______________ Weight ____________

Birthmark, if any _________________________ Zodiac Sign ____________

Health Record

Age	Date	Length	Weight
First week			
Second week			
Third week			
First month			
Second month			
Third month			
Fourth month			
Fifth month			
Sixth month			

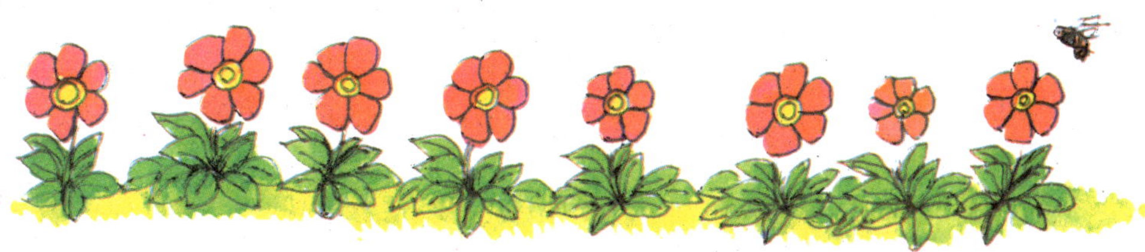

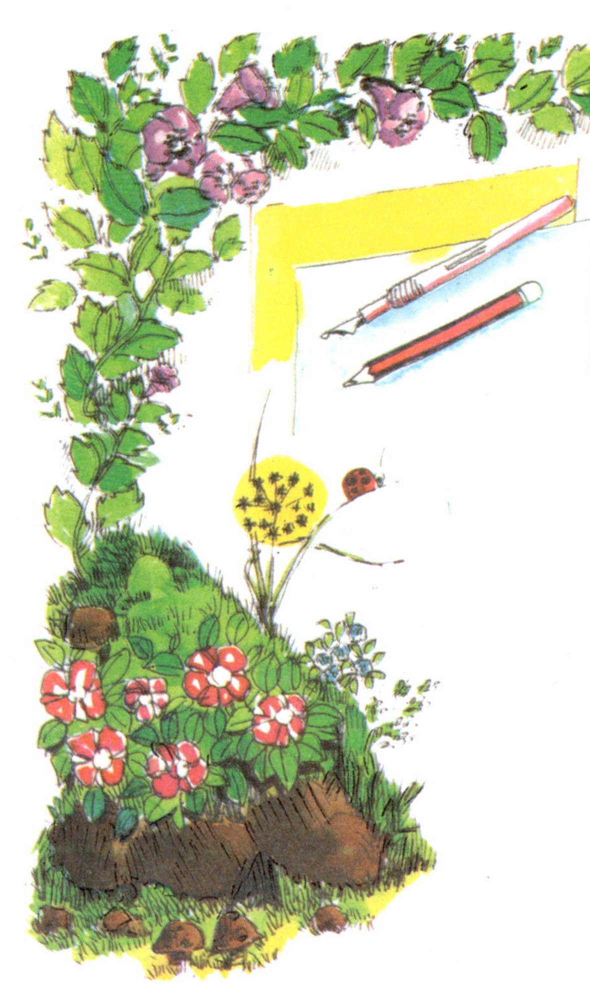

Blessings/Congratulations

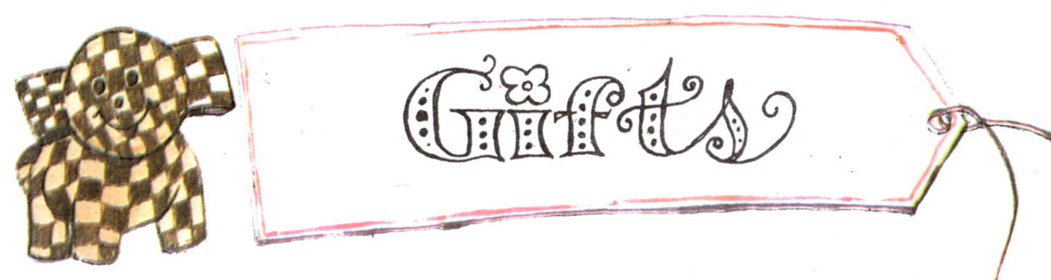

Guests	Gifts

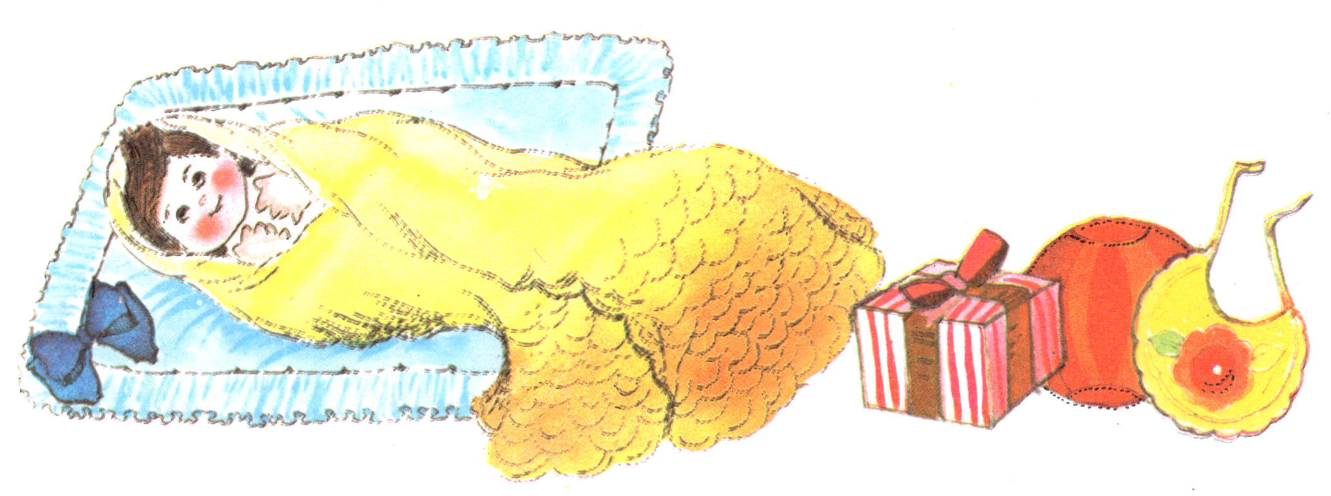

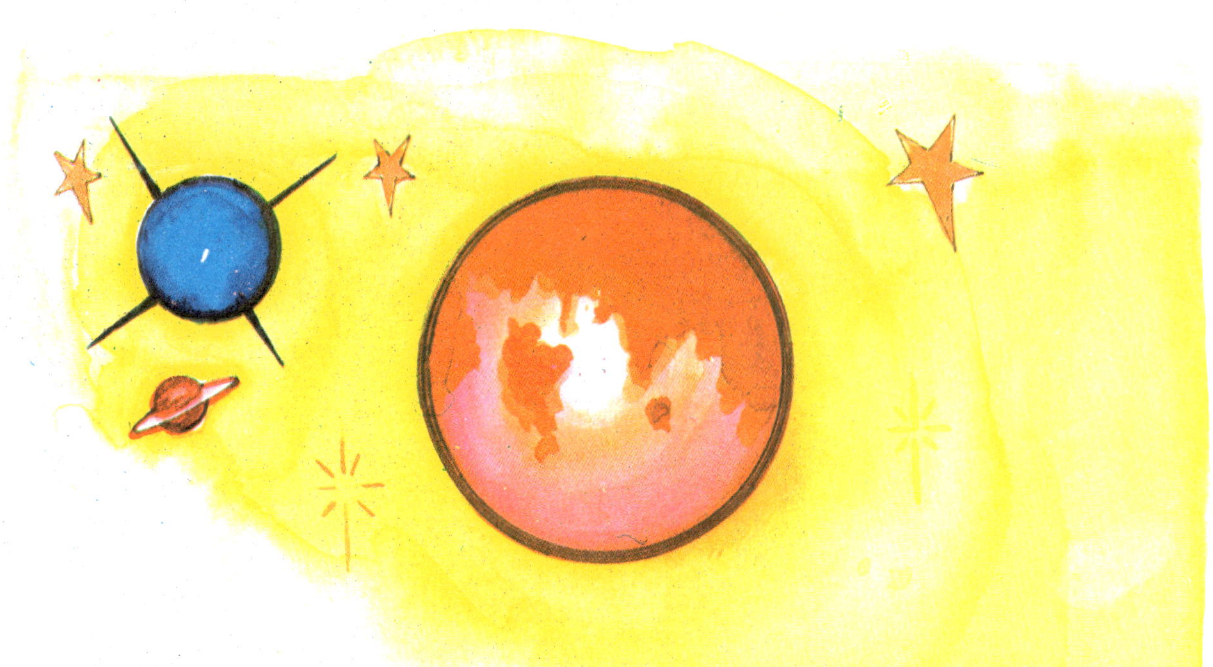

Significant Happenings

(In family. In India and Abroad)

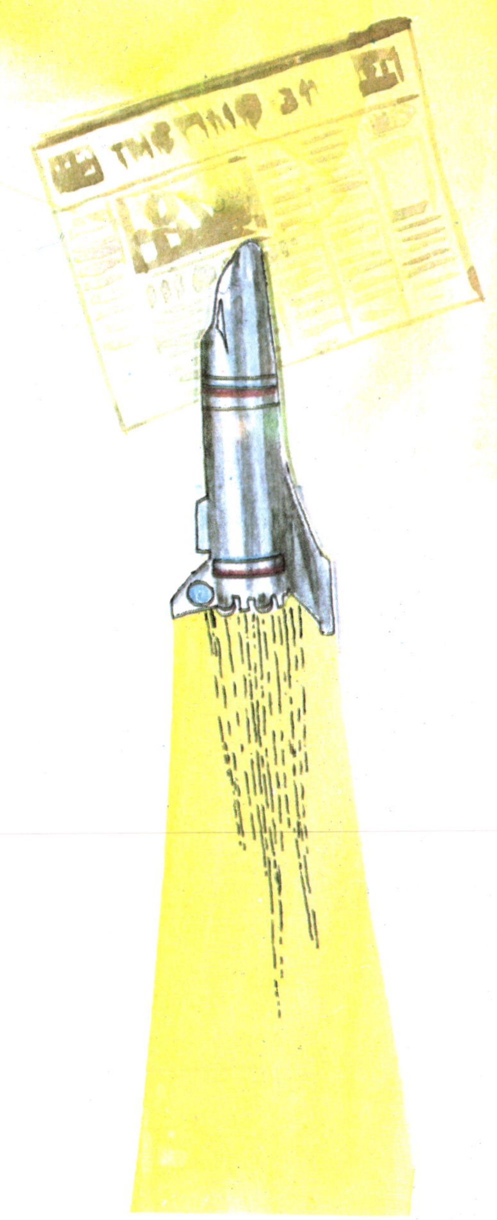

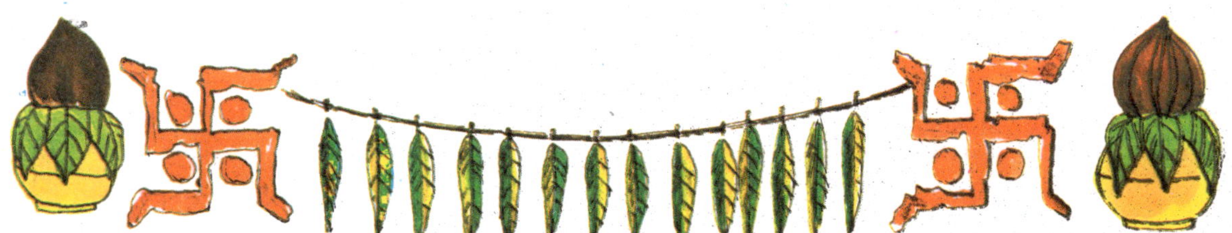

Sixth-Day-Bath

Photograph

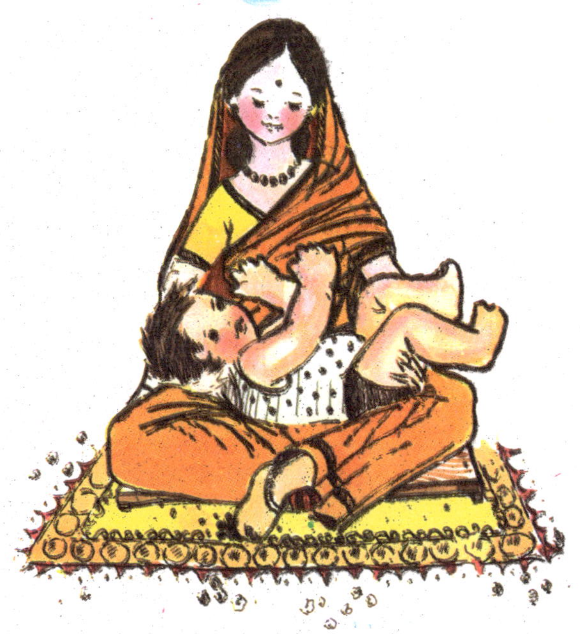

Date ______________________

Place ______________________

Priest ______________________

Horoscope

Time of Sunrise

Birth time after Sunrise

Rashi (Chandra)

Varna

Yoni

Gana

Lord of Chandra Rashi

Nadi

Year

Month

Paksha

Date

Day

Constellation

Yog

Duration of the day

Rashi

Name according to Chandra Rashi

Made by

Naming ceremony

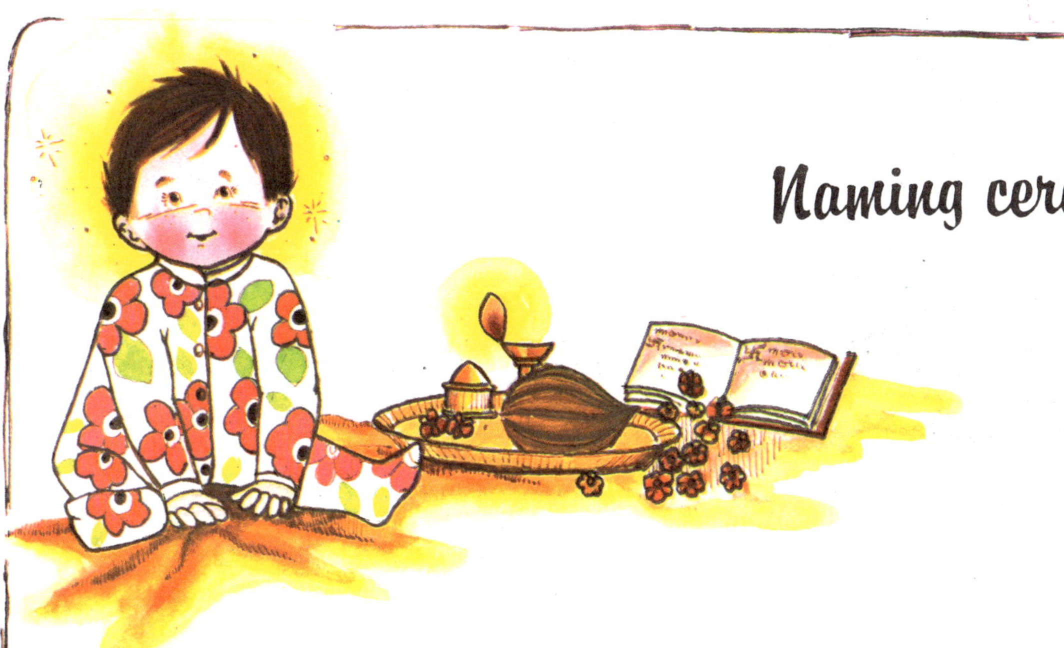

Name Suggested by:

Mother
Father
Grand-parents
Uncle/Aunt
Brother/Sister
Friends

Affix Photograph

Selected name

Date

Pet name

Place

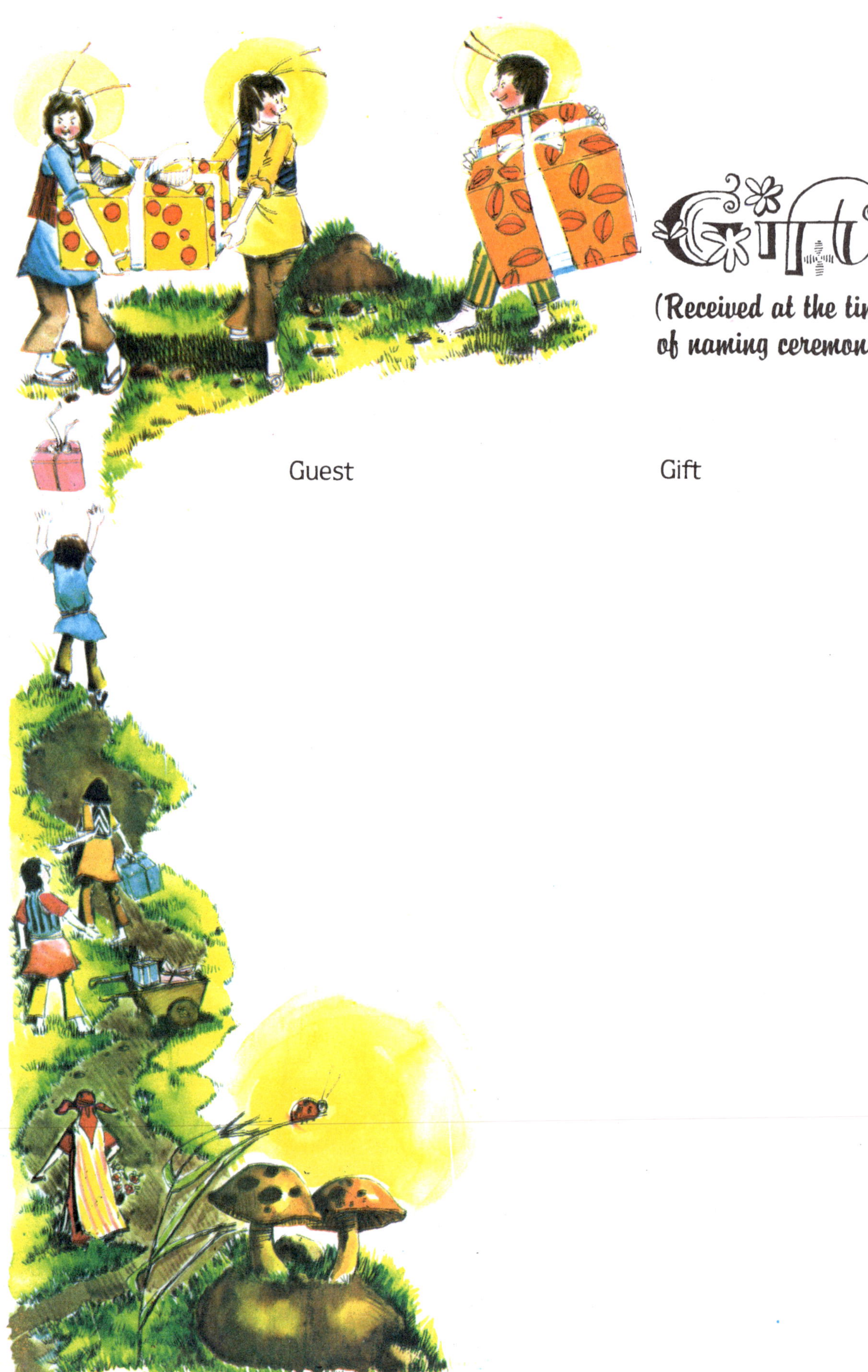

Gifts

(Received at the time of naming ceremony)

Guest	Gift

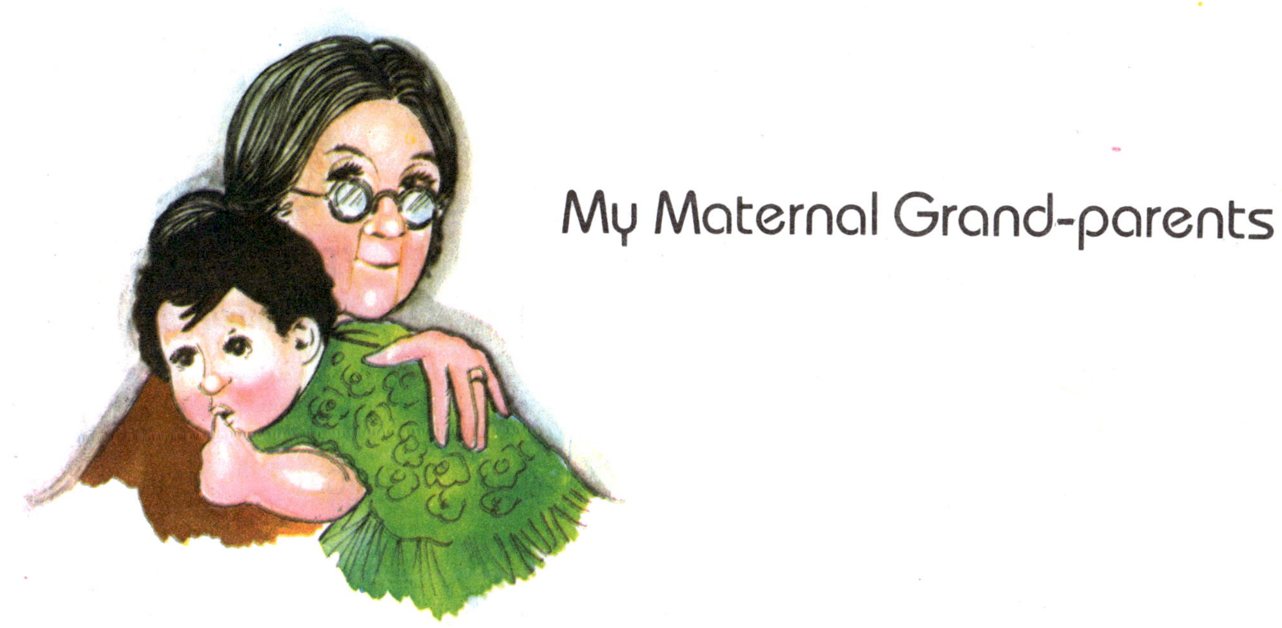

My Maternal Grand-parents

Affix Photograph

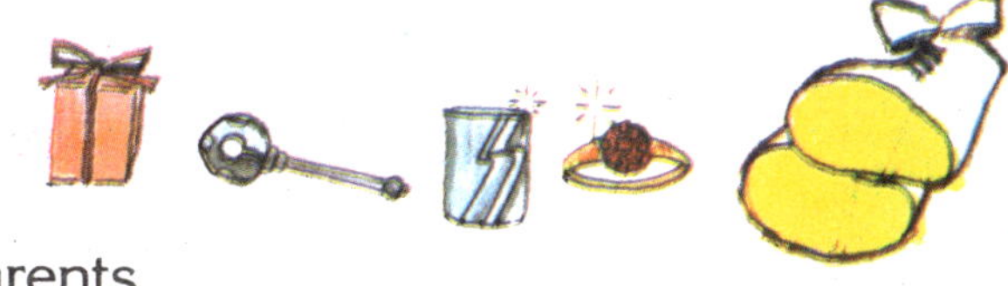

Gifts received from maternal Grand-parents

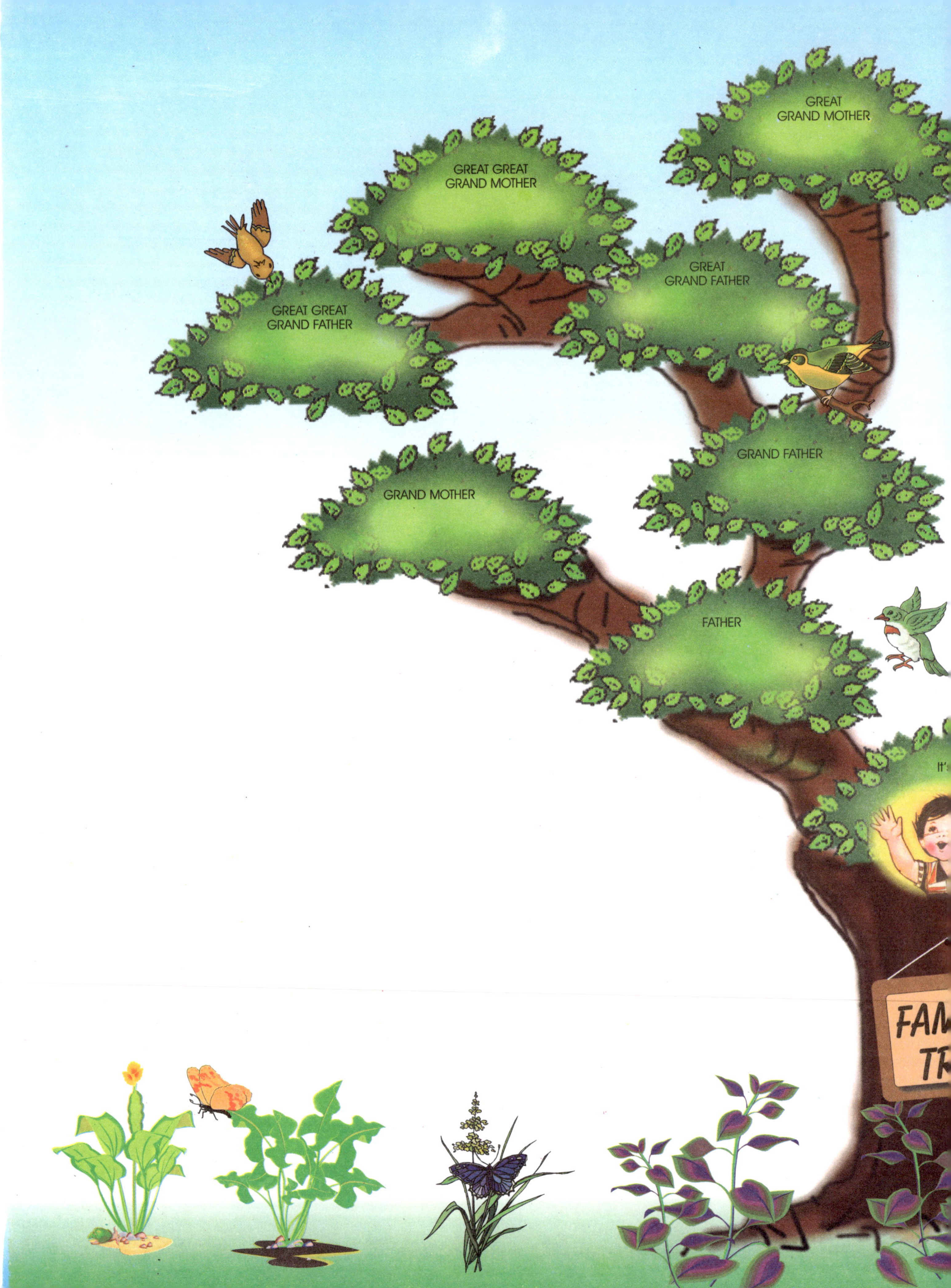
GREAT GREAT
GRAND MOTHER
GREAT
GRAND MOTHER
GREAT GREAT
GRAND FATHER
GREAT
GRAND FATHER
GRAND FATHER
GRAND MOTHER
FATHER

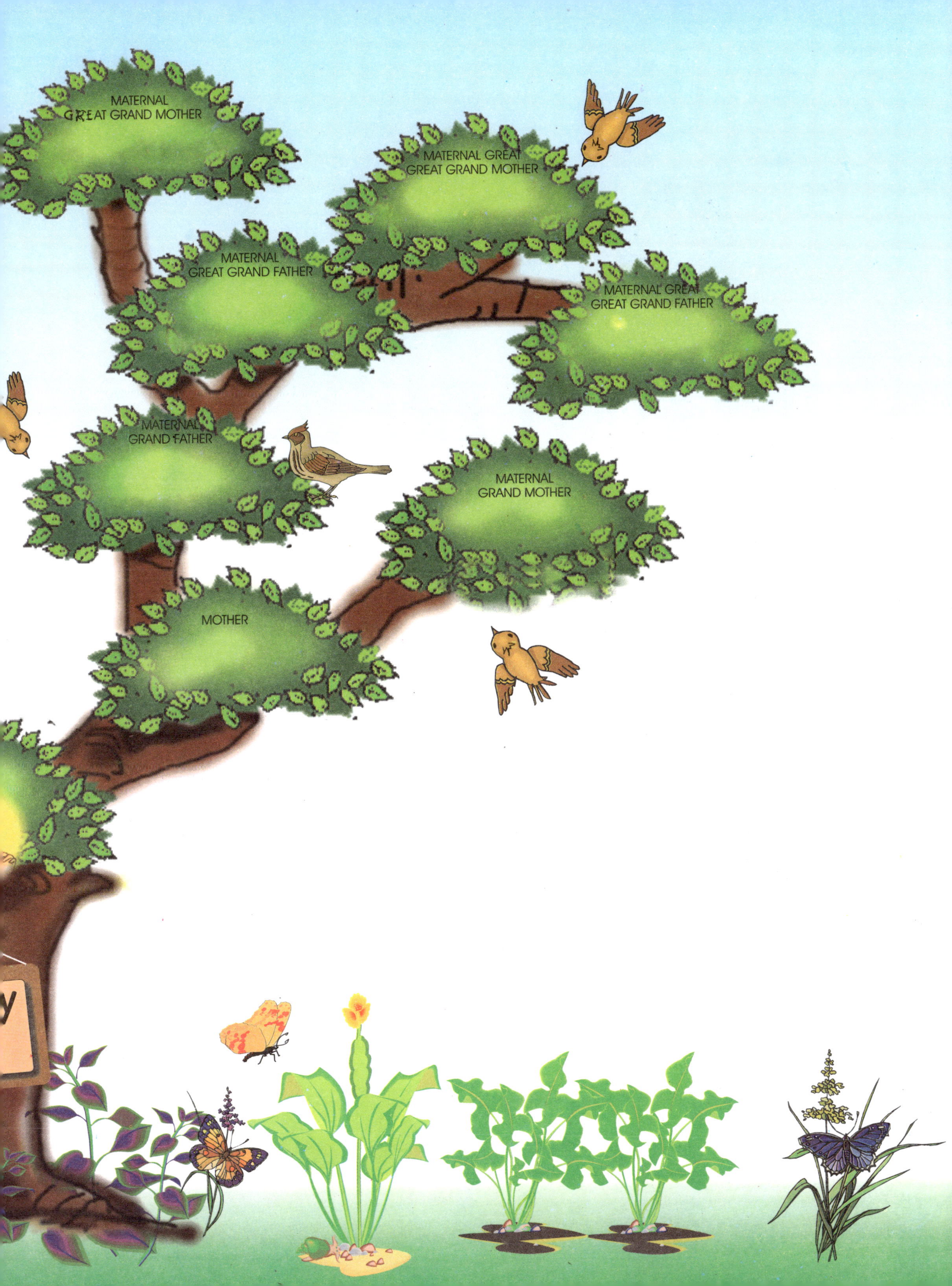
MATERNAL
GREAT GRAND MOTHER
MATERNAL GREAT
GREAT GRAND MOTHER
MATERNAL
GREAT GRAND FATHER
MATERNAL GREAT
GREAT GRAND FATHER
MATERNAL
GRAND FATHER
MATERNAL
GRAND MOTHER
MOTHER

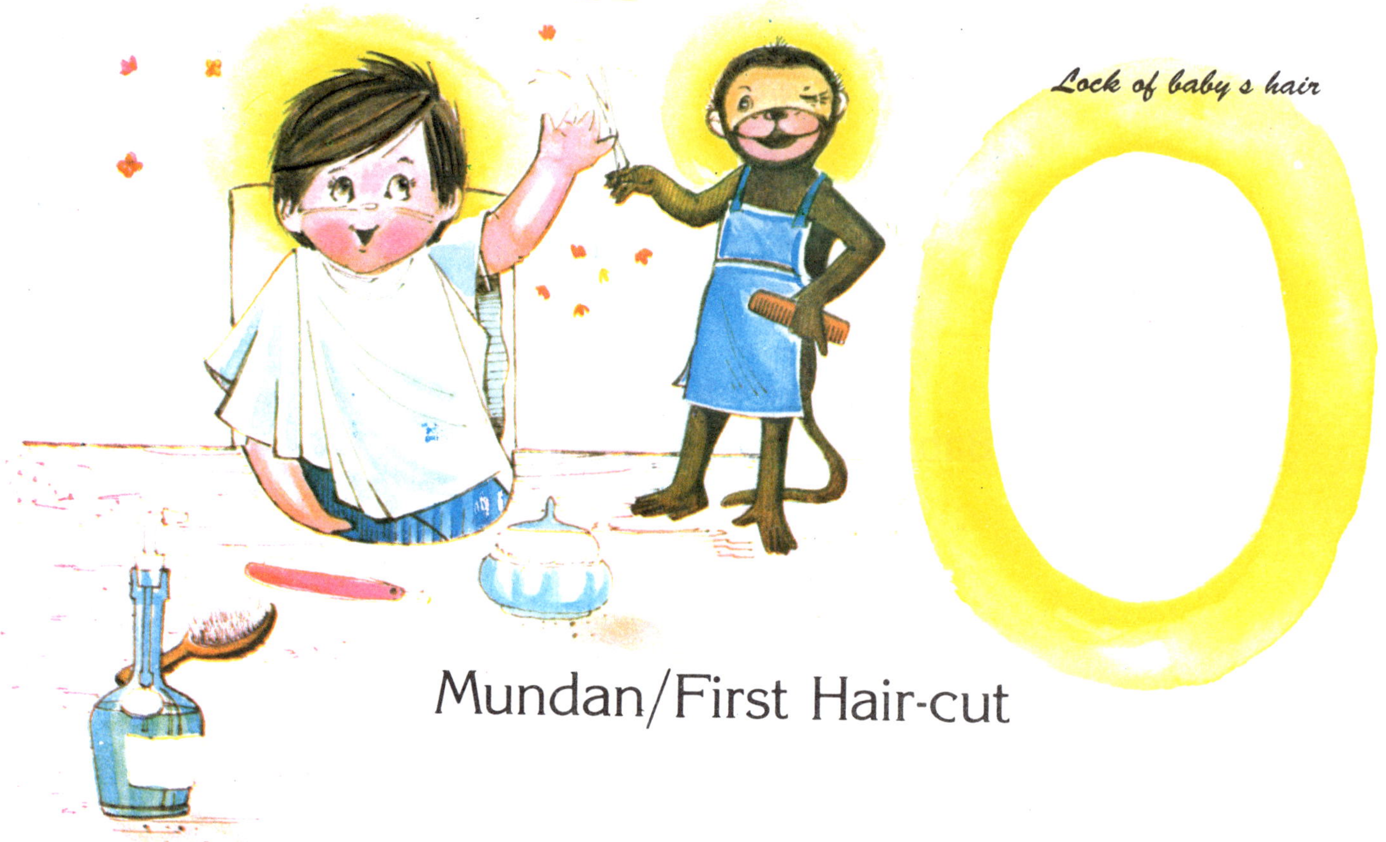

Mundan/First Hair-cut

Affix Photograph

Date ______ ______ Place ____________________

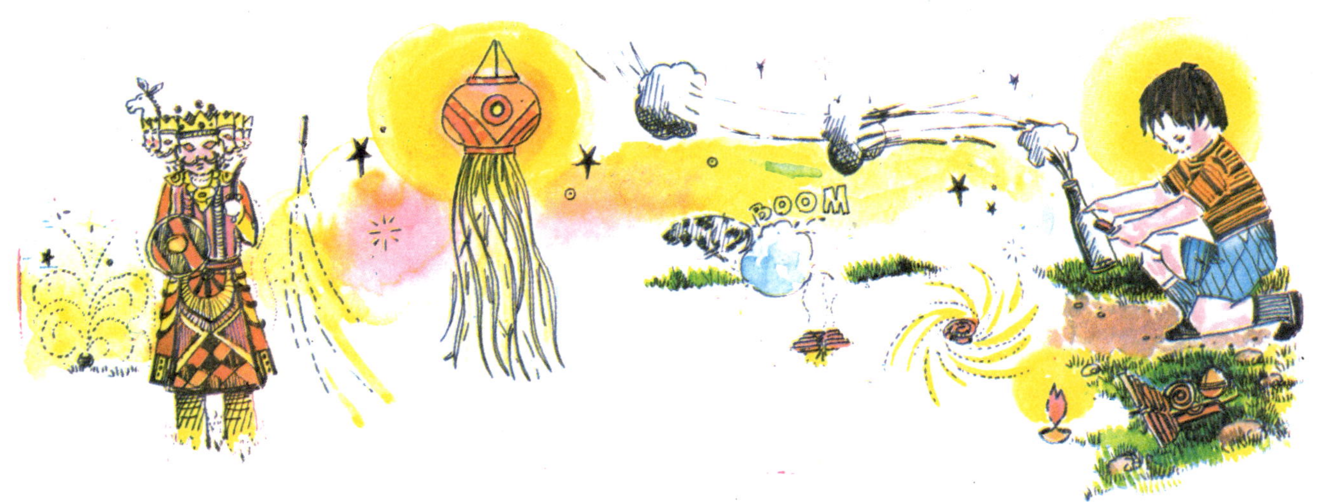

Baby's First Festivals

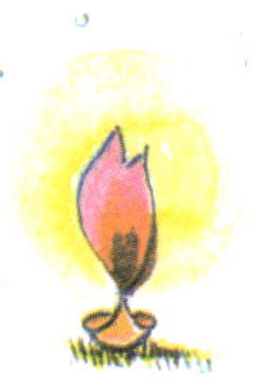

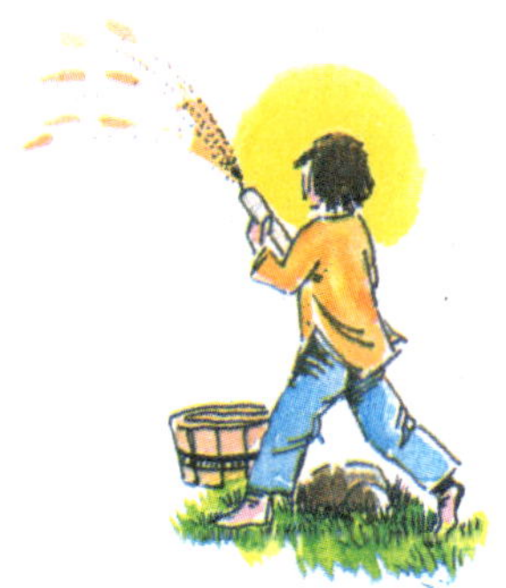

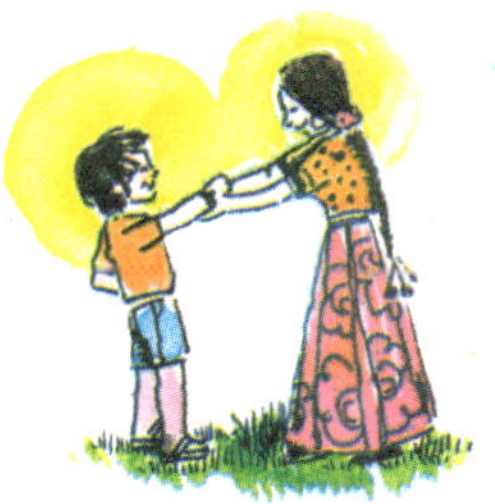

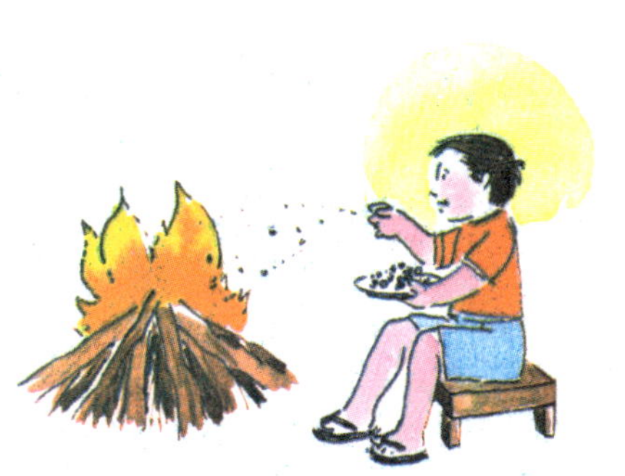

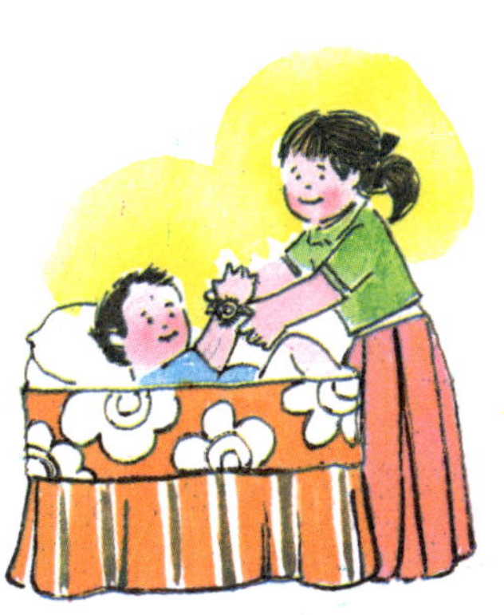

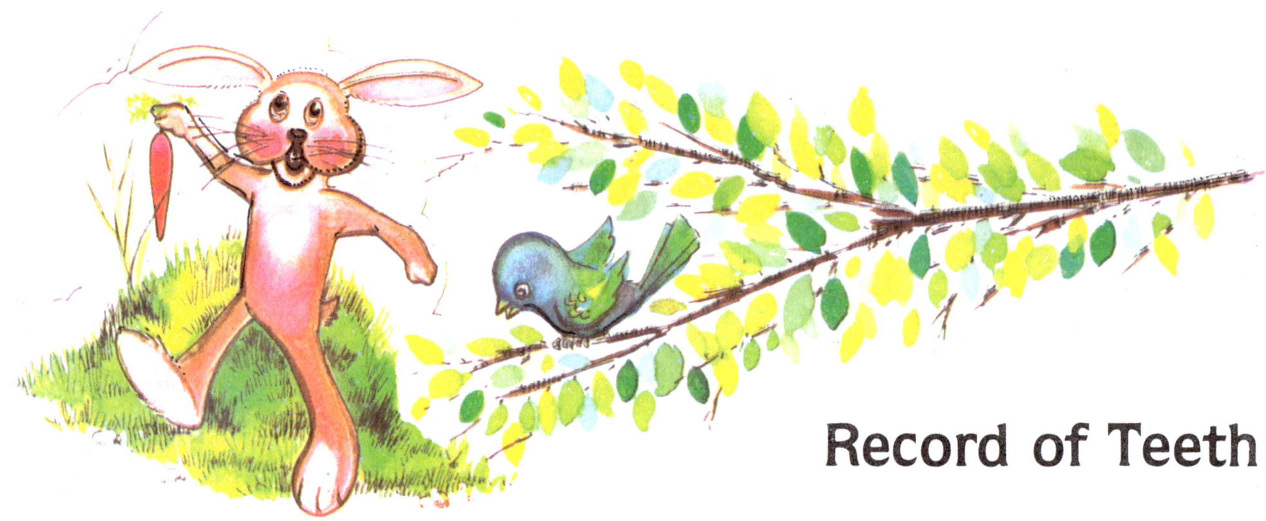

Record of Teeth

Upper Jaw

Date

Date

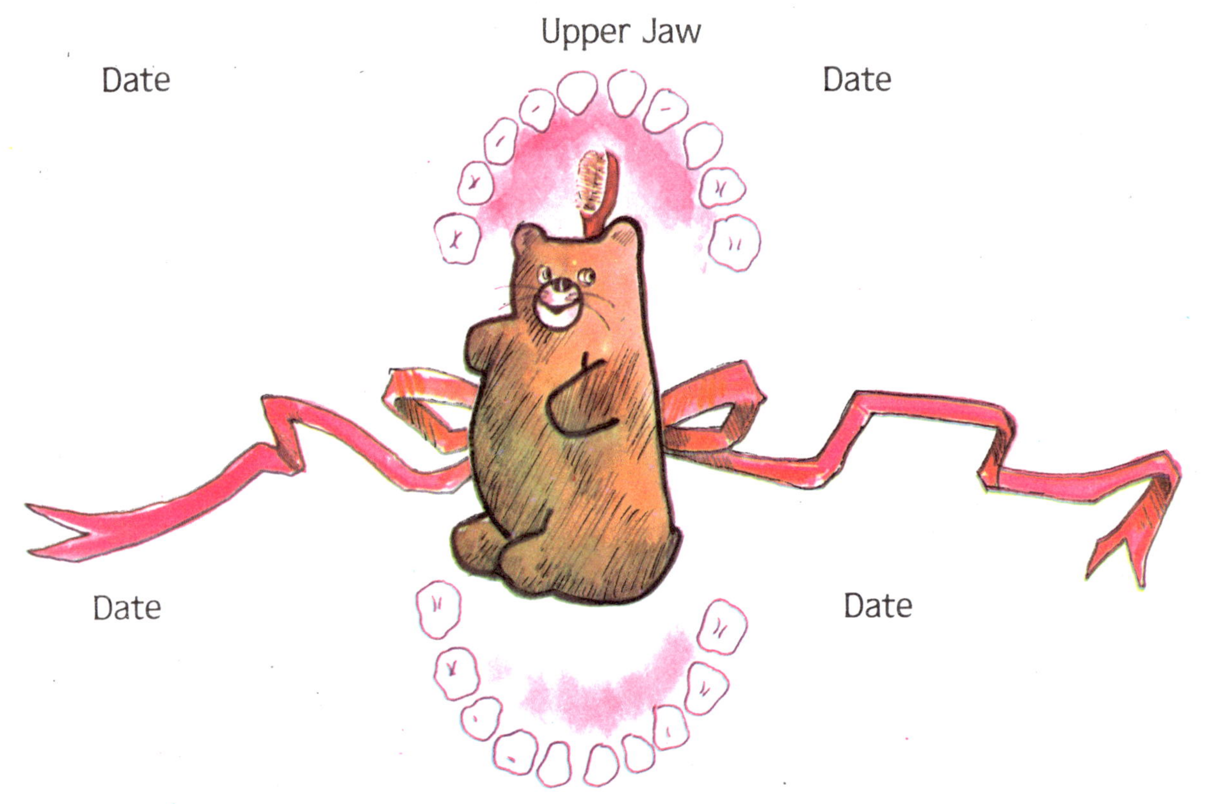

Date

Date

Lower Jaw

Other details about baby's health

Vaccination Table

Disease	Vaccine/ Medicine	Date of First Vaccination	Name of Doctor/ Hospital	Date of Second Vaccination	Date of Third Vaccination
1. Tuberculosis	B.C.G.				
2. Whooping Cough, Tetanus and Diphtheria	Triple Antigen				
3. Polio	Polio-drops				
4. Typhoid	Vaccine				
5. Measles	Vaccine				
6. Hepatitis B	Vaccine				
7. Measles, Mumps, Rubella	M.M.R. Vaccine				

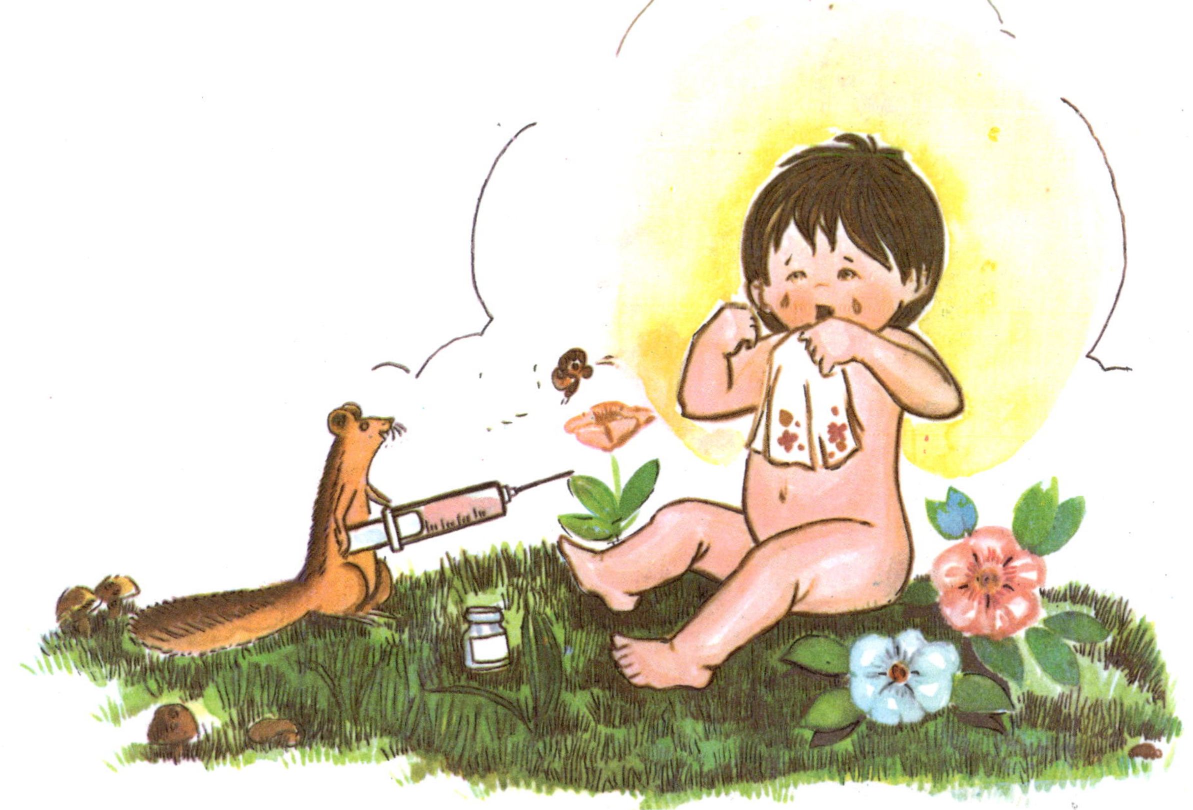

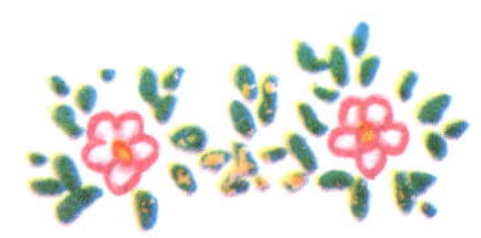

Milestones of Baby's Growth

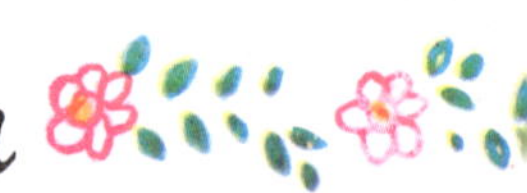

Affix Photograph

Affix Photograph

Date ____________________

Date ____________________

SEE, NOW I CAN SIT

I'VE LEARNT CRAWLING TOO

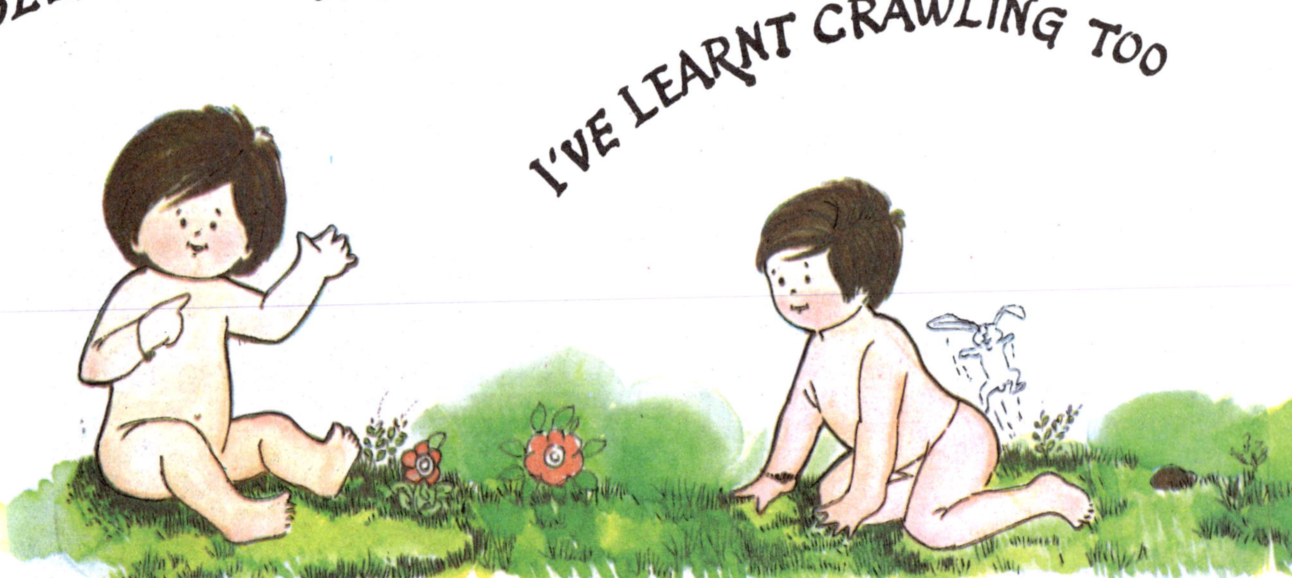

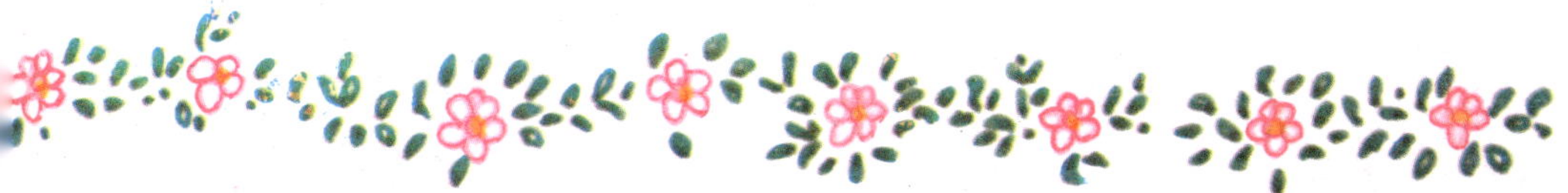

Affix Photograph

Affix Photograph

Date ____________________

Date ____________________

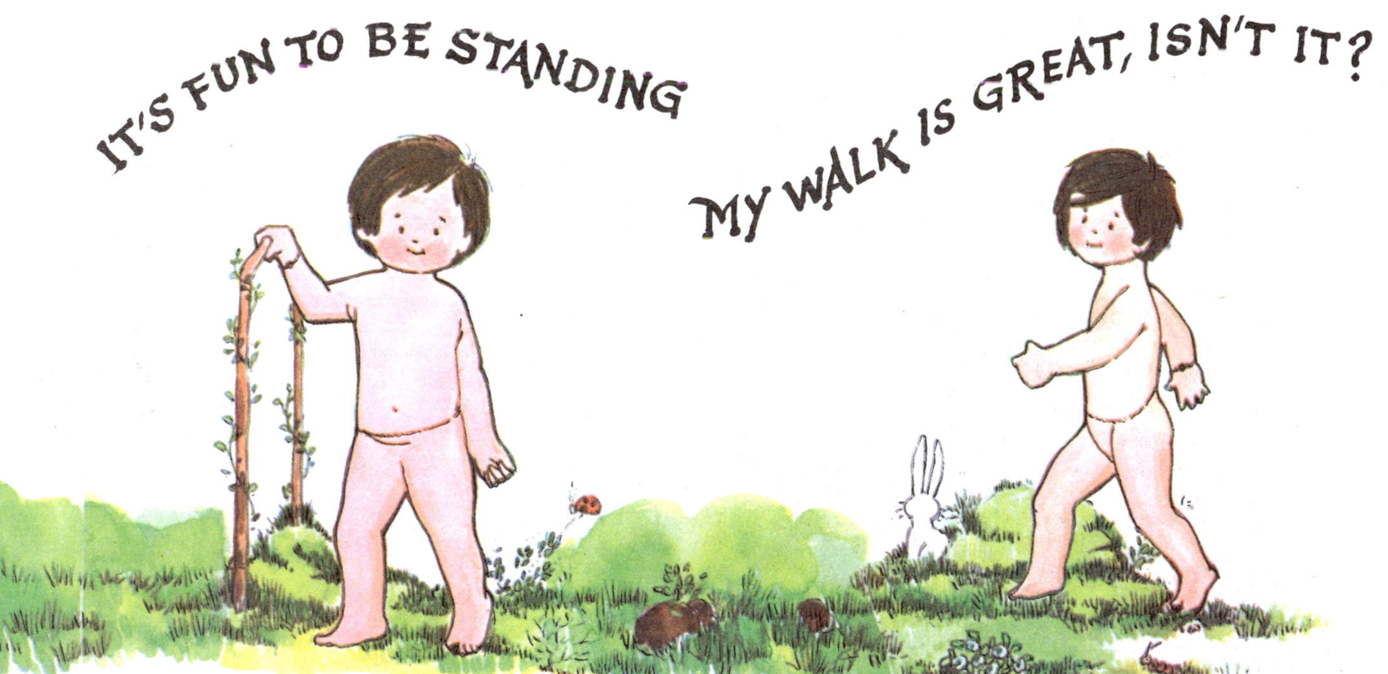

My First Birthday

Affix Photograph

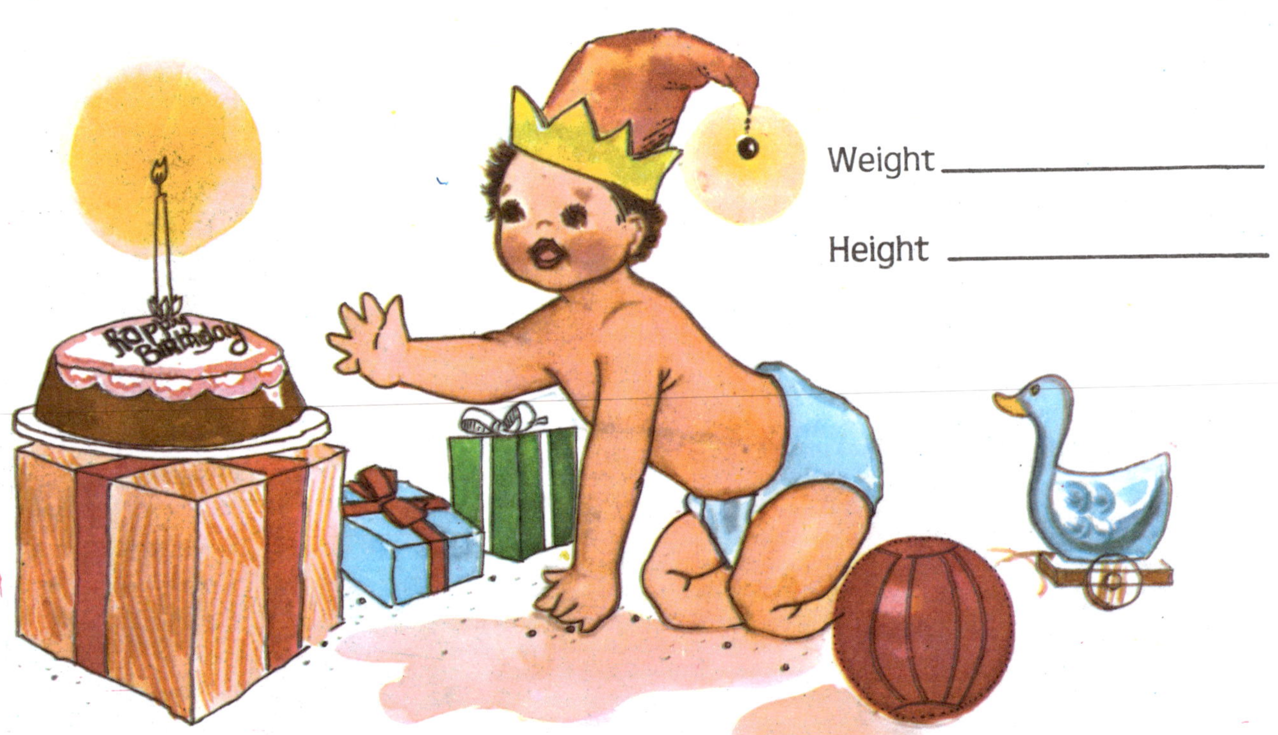

Weight ______________________

Height ______________________

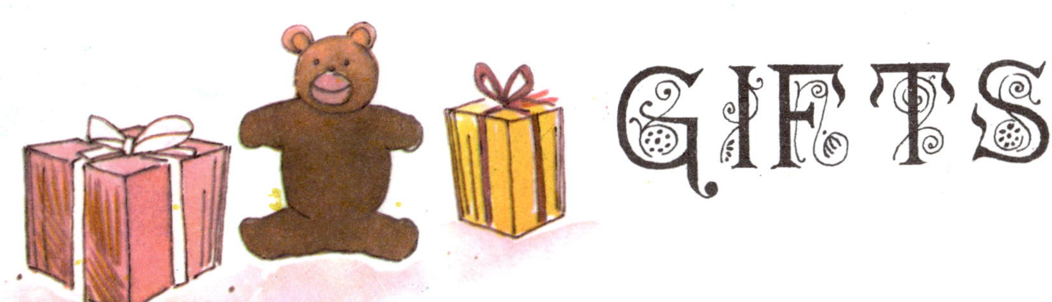

GIFTS

Guests

Gifts

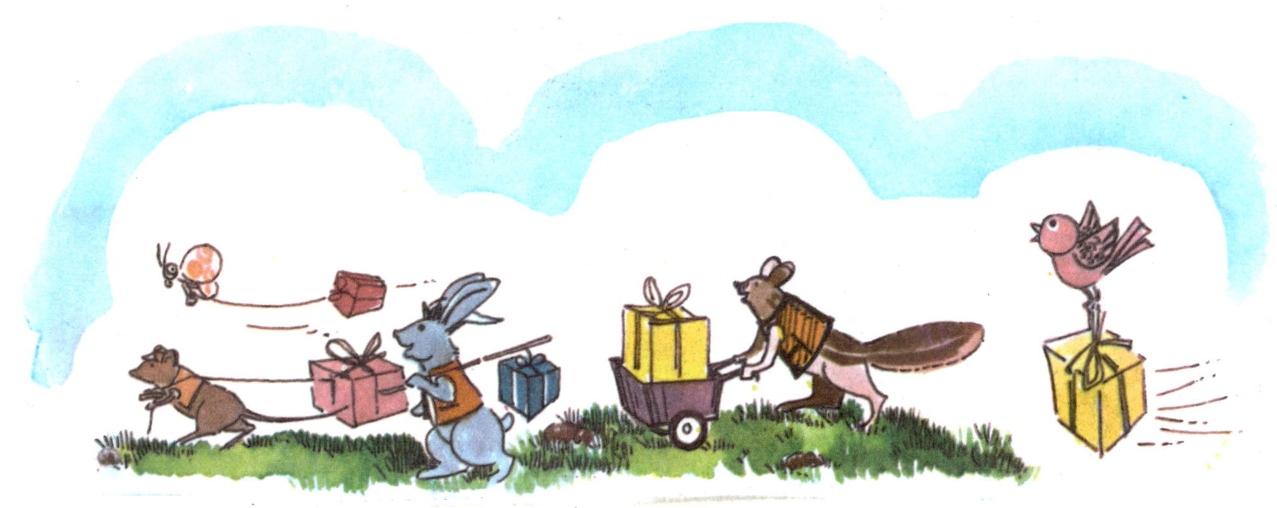

My Second Birthday

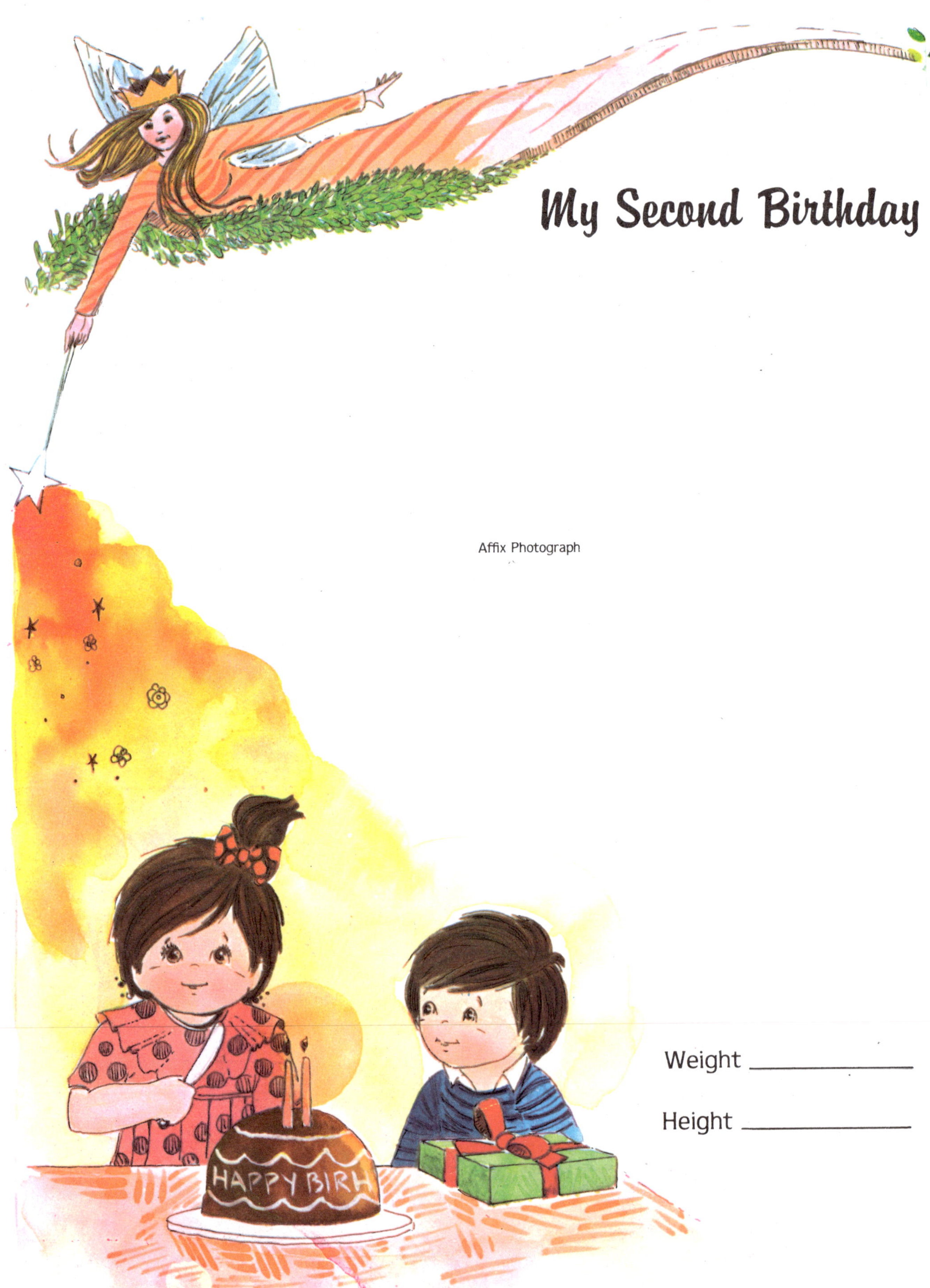

Affix Photograph

Weight ______________

Height ______________

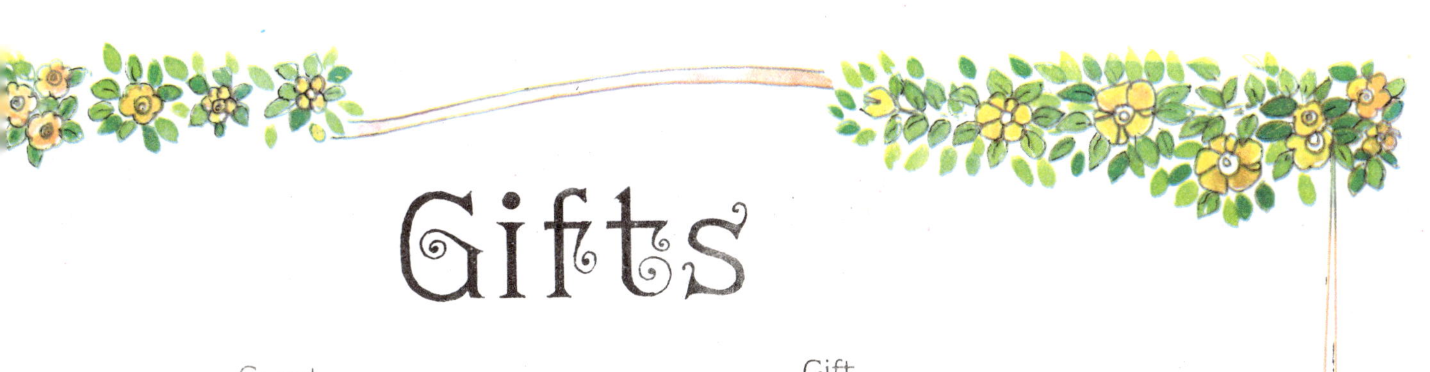

Gifts

Guest	Gift

My Third Birthday

Affix Photograph

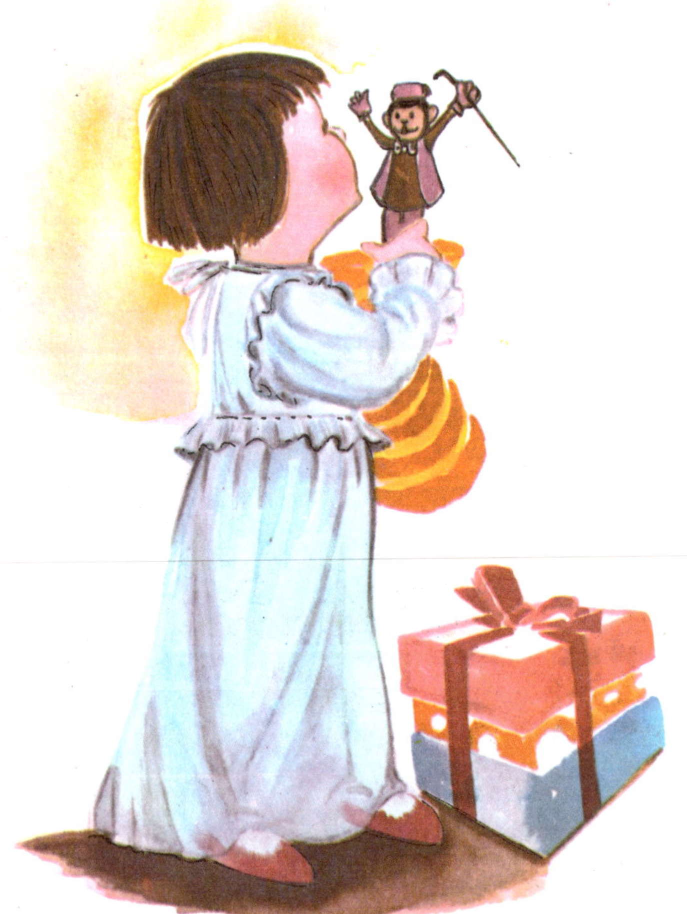

Height ______________________

Weight ______________________

Now starts my Schooling

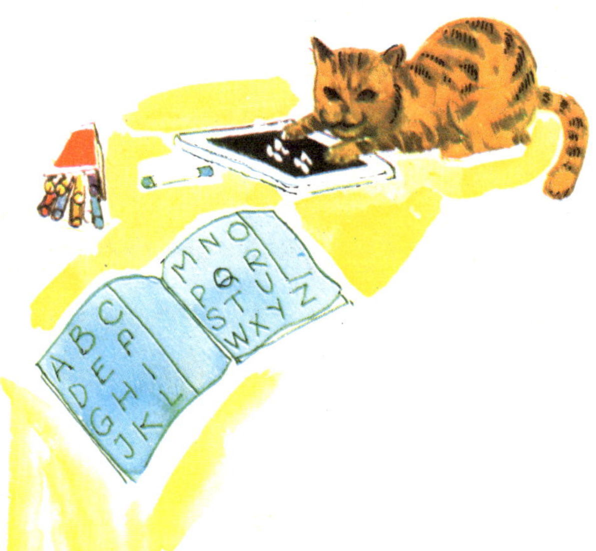

Date of admission ____________ Class ____________

Teacher ______________________________

School ______________________________

Affix Photograph

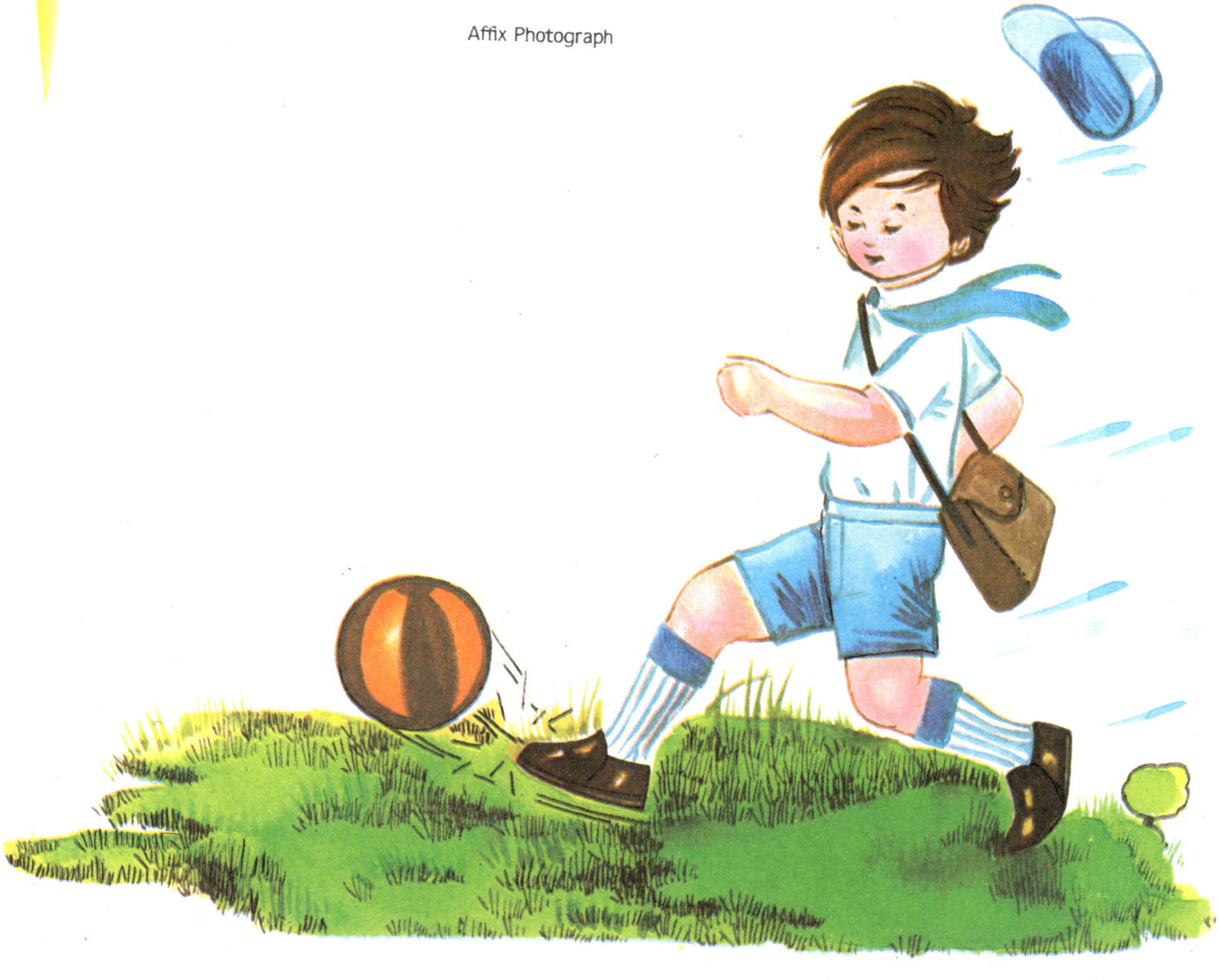

My Fourth Birthday

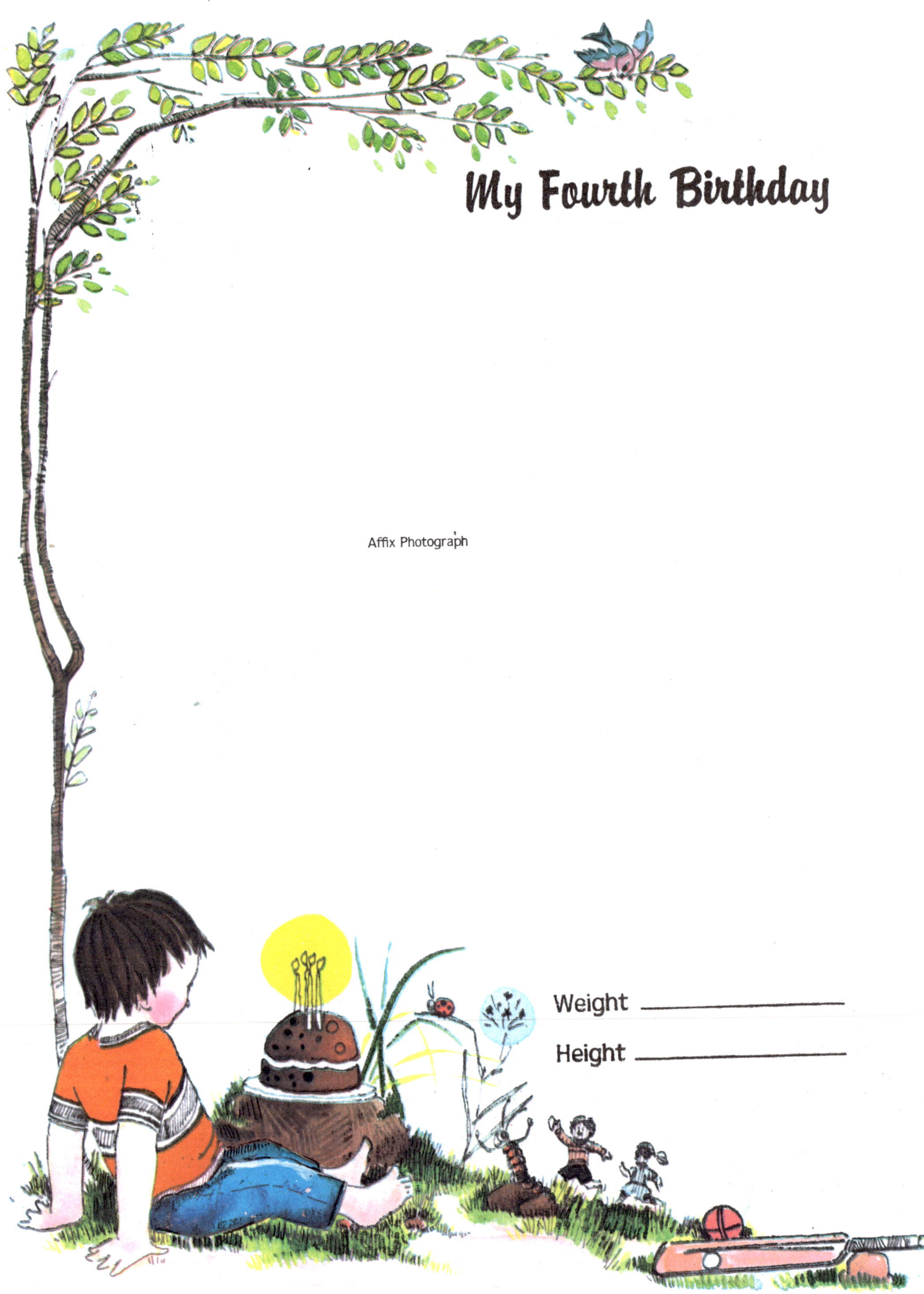

Affix Photograph

Weight ______________

Height ______________

My Fifth Birthday

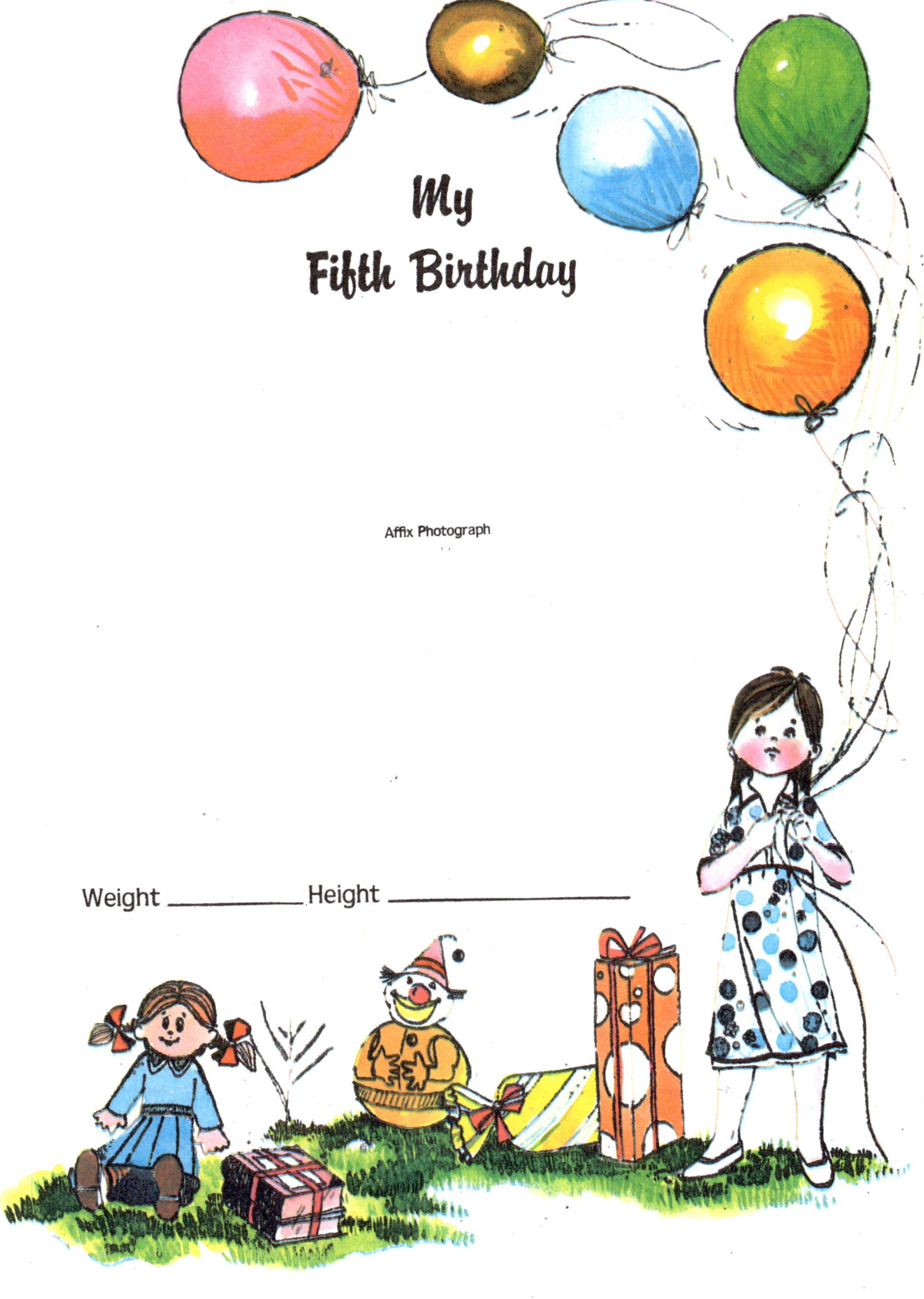

Affix Photograph

Weight ______________ Height ________________________

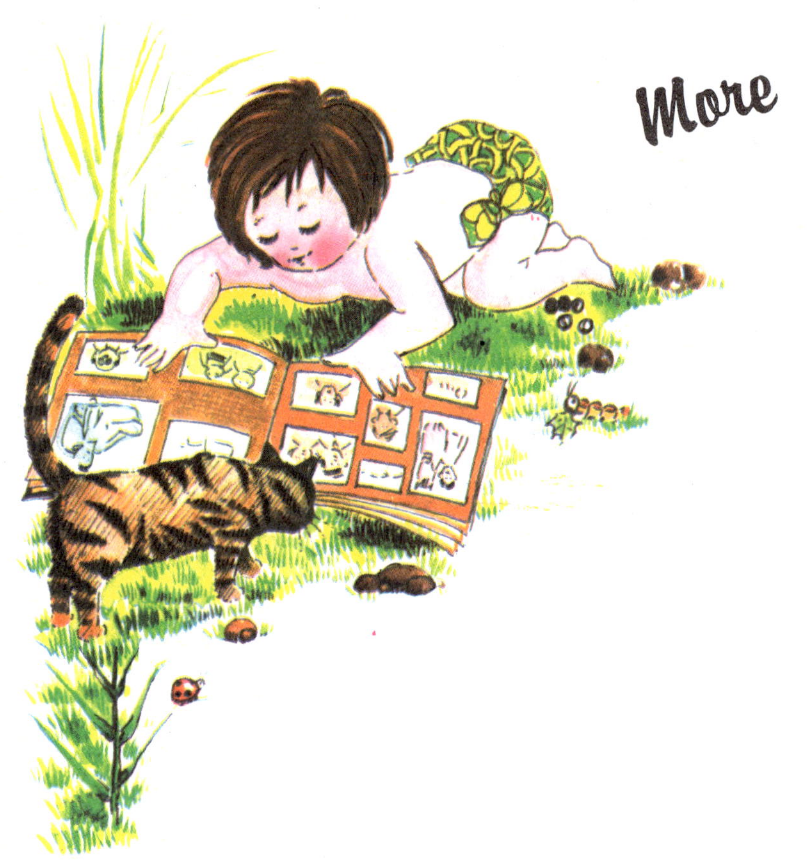

More photographs of

Affix Photograph

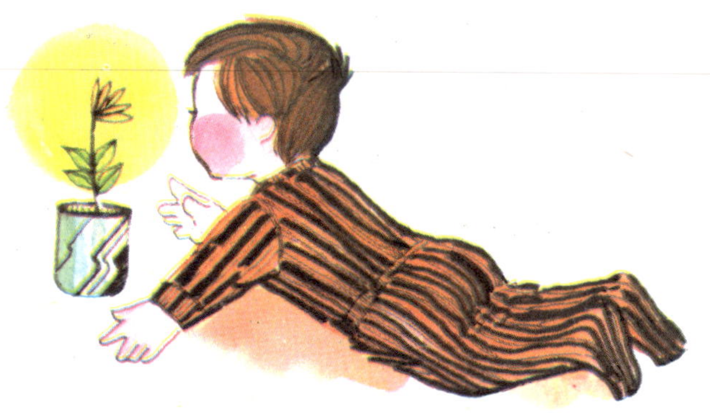

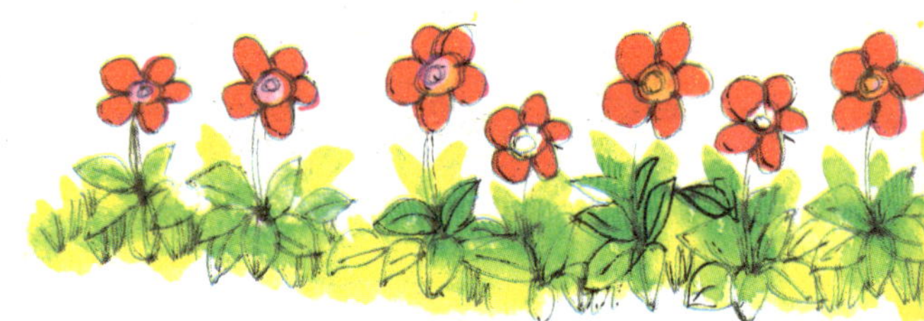

My/baby's childhood

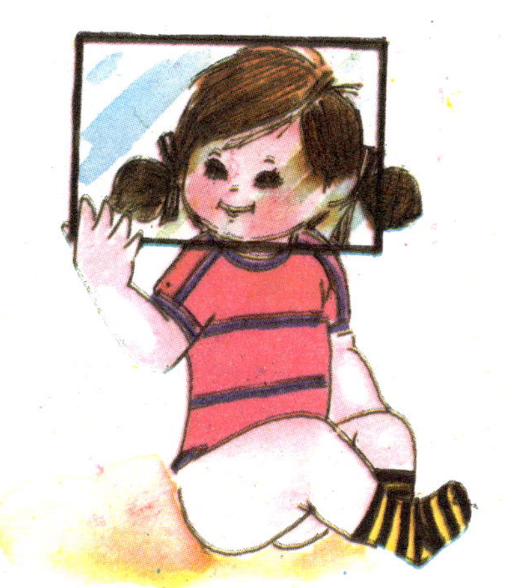

Affix Photograph

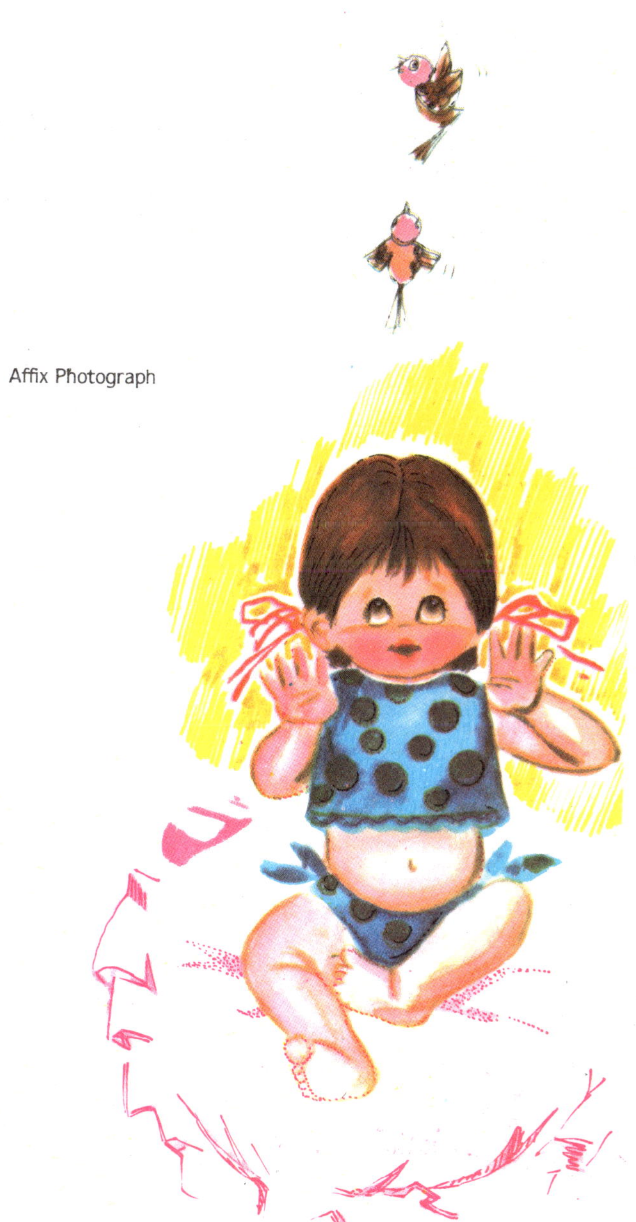

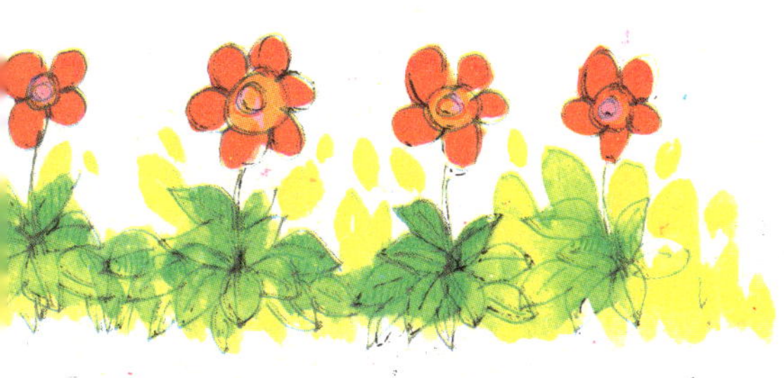

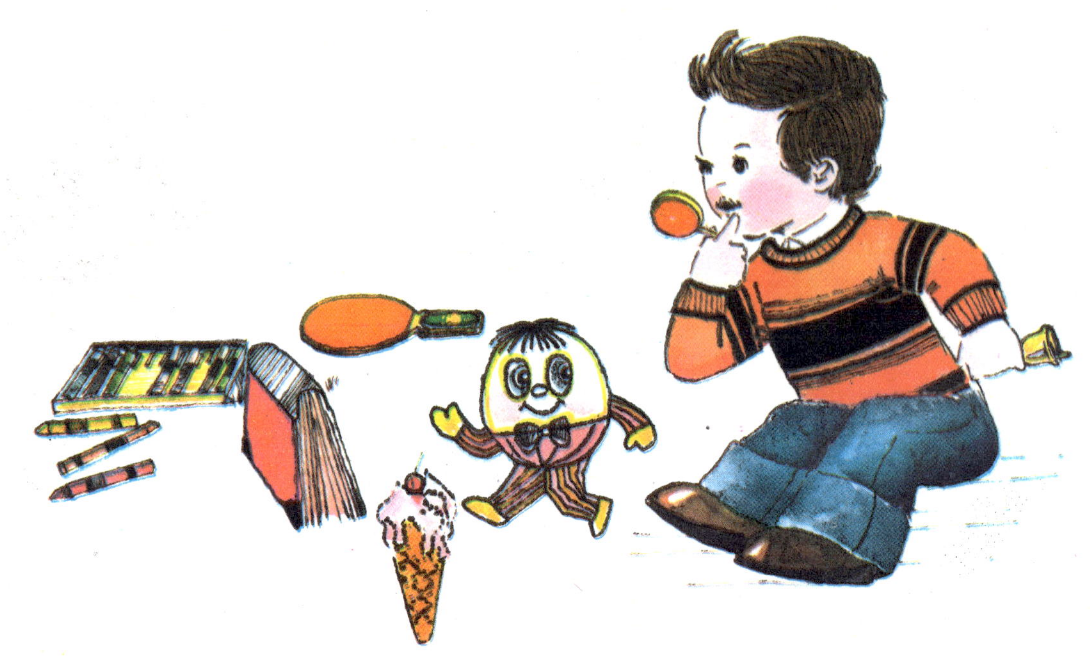

What a wonderful world of toys!

(My Hobbies and Interests)

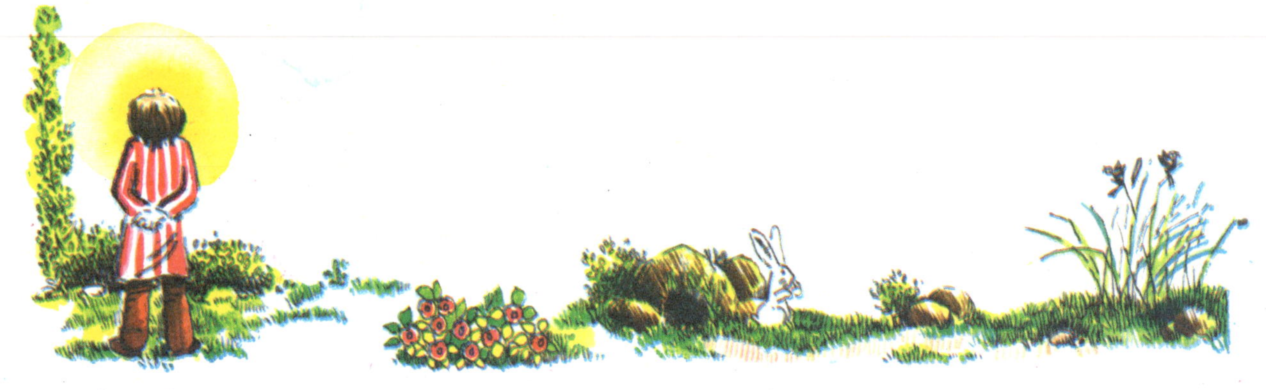

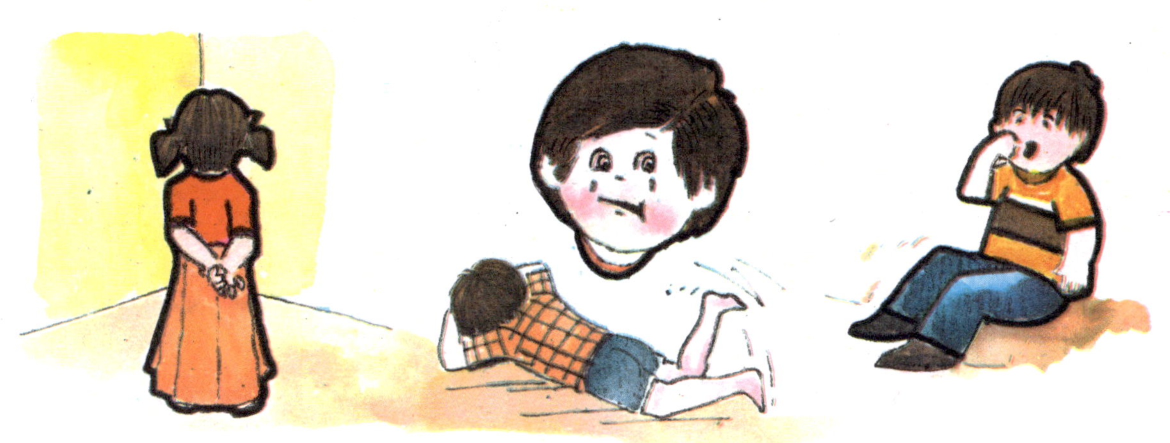

I'll weep and cry, but have my way---

(Stubborn and naughty actions)

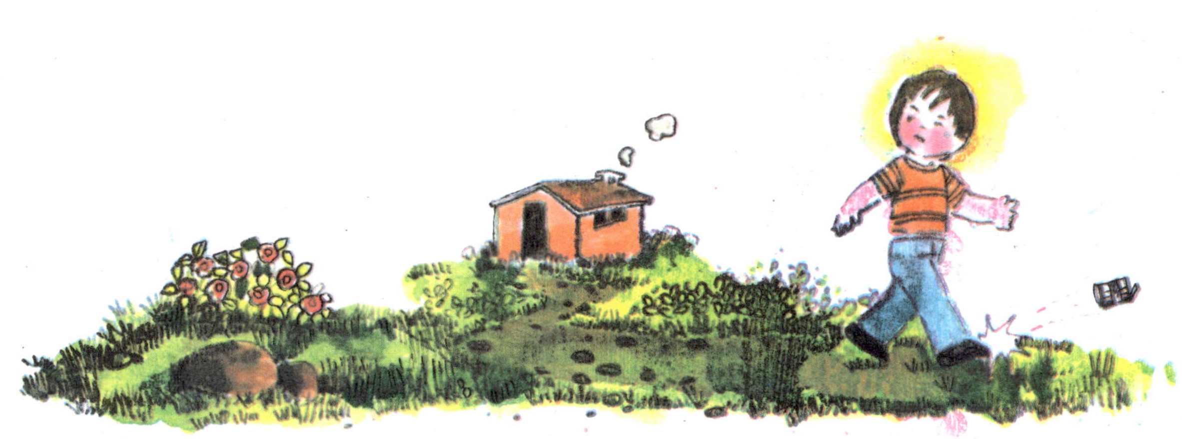

Significant Events during Childhood

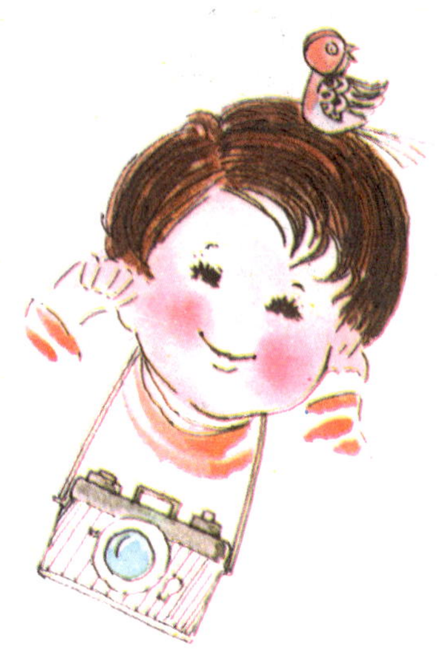

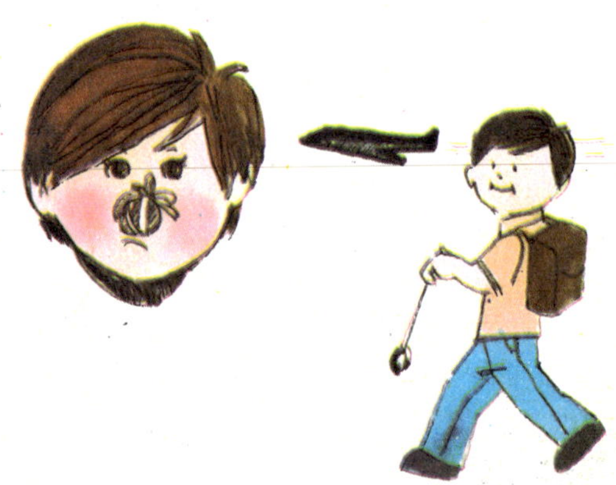

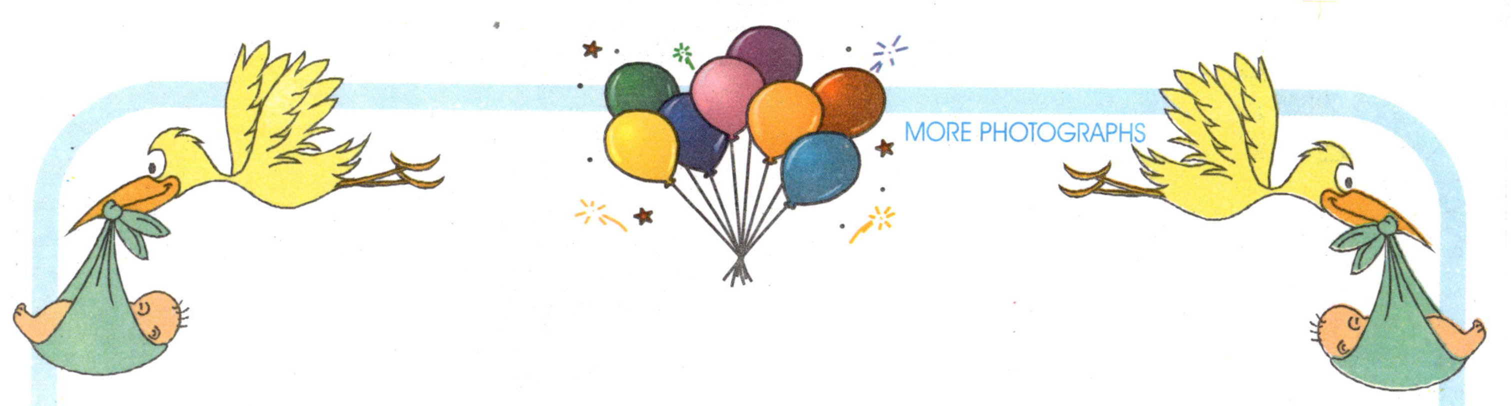
MORE PHOTOGRAPHS

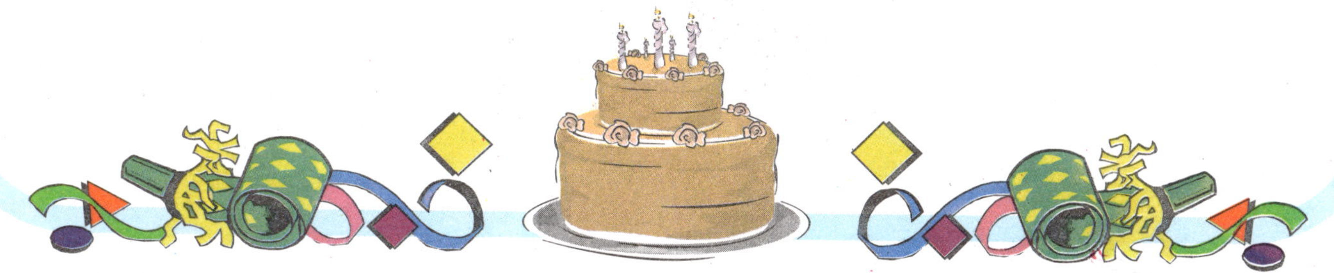

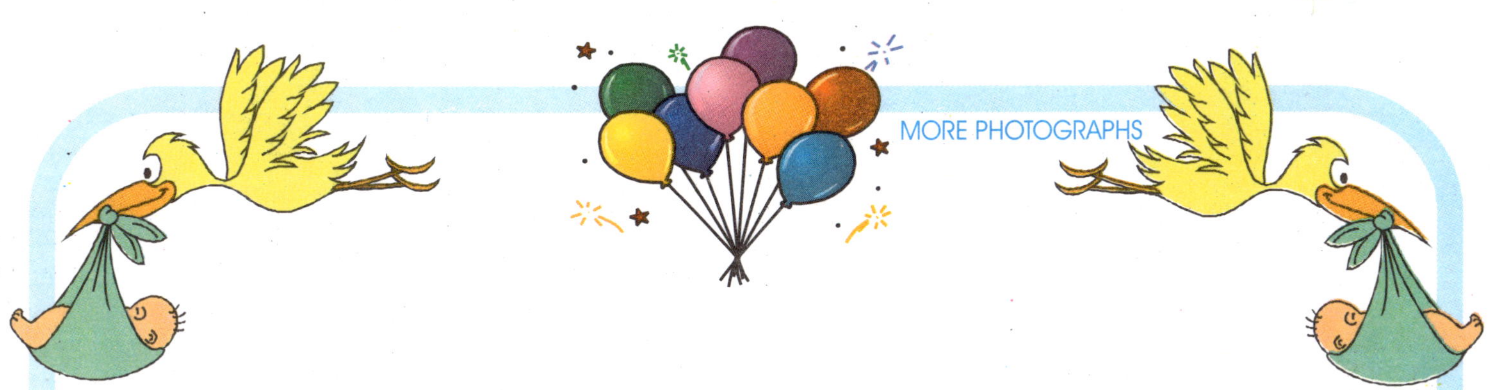
MORE PHOTOGRAPHS

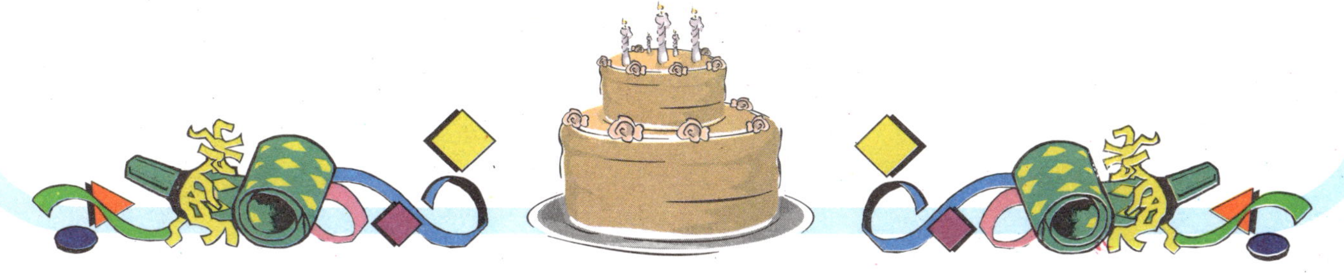

MORE PHOTOGRAPHS

MORE PHOTOGRAPHS

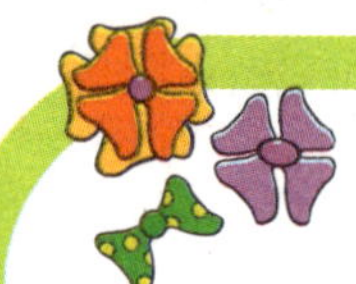

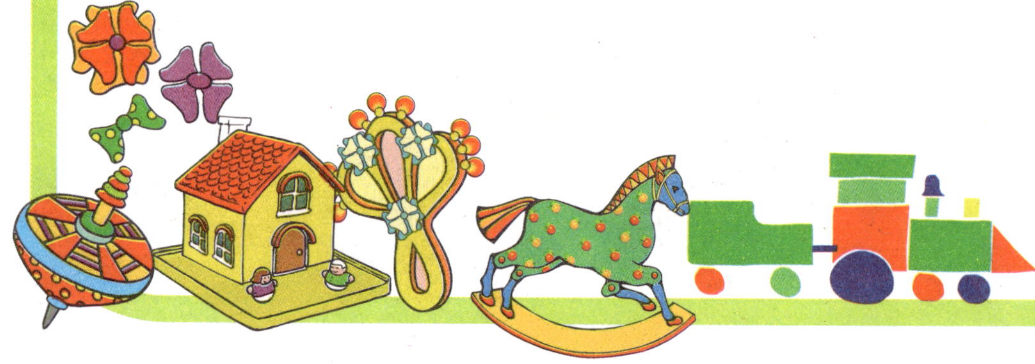

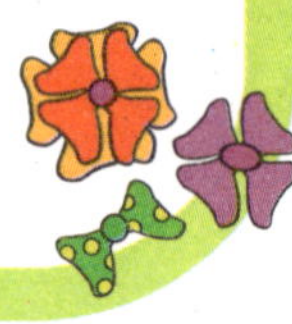

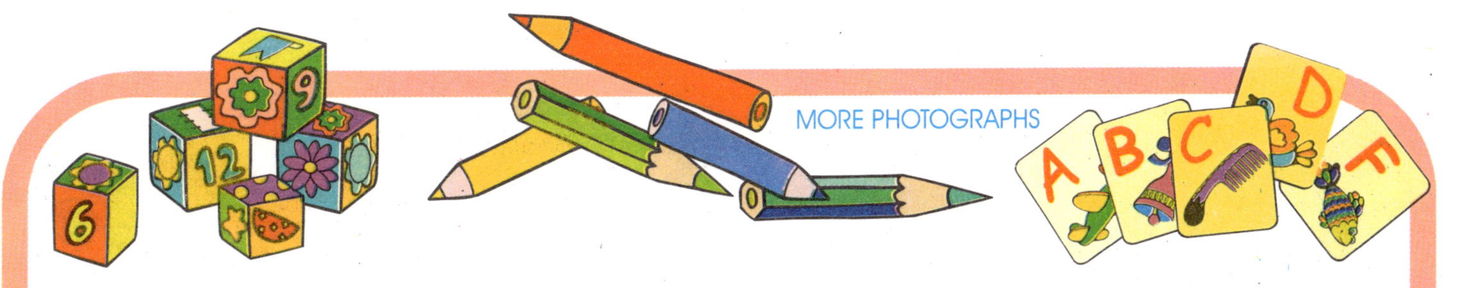
MORE PHOTOGRAPHS

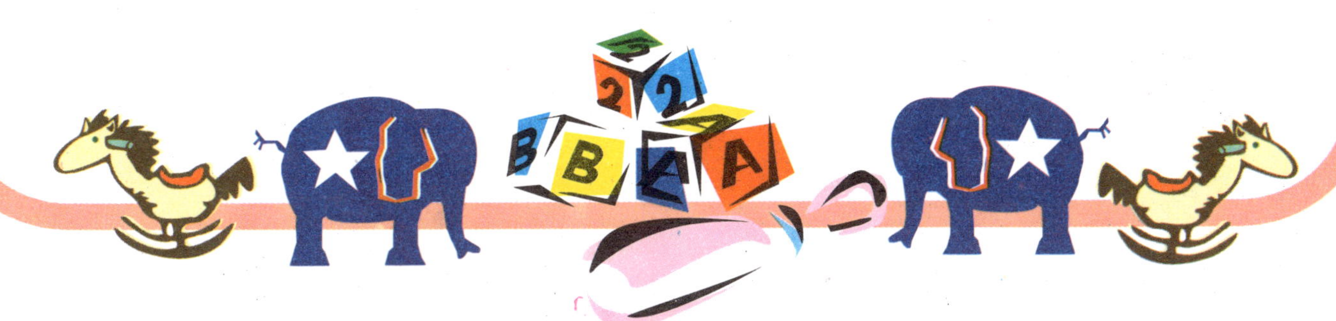

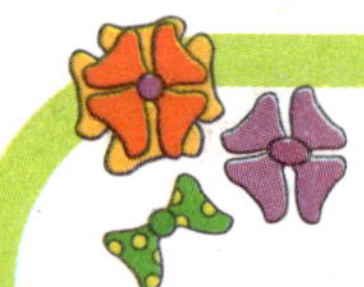

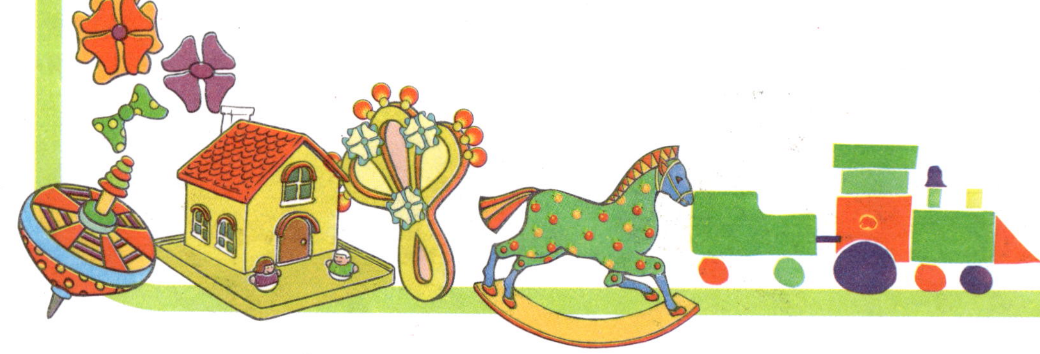

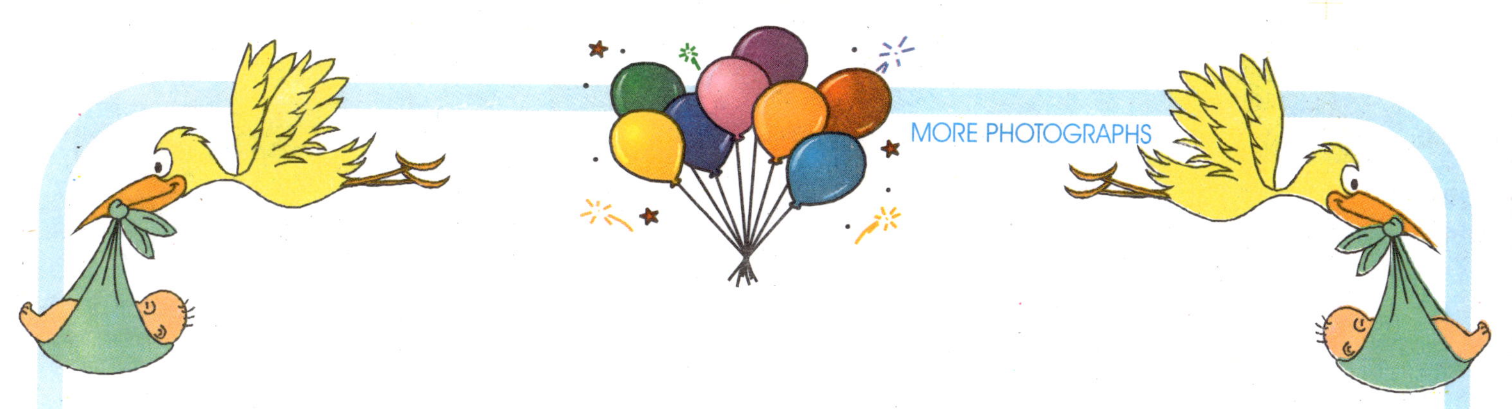
MORE PHOTOGRAPHS

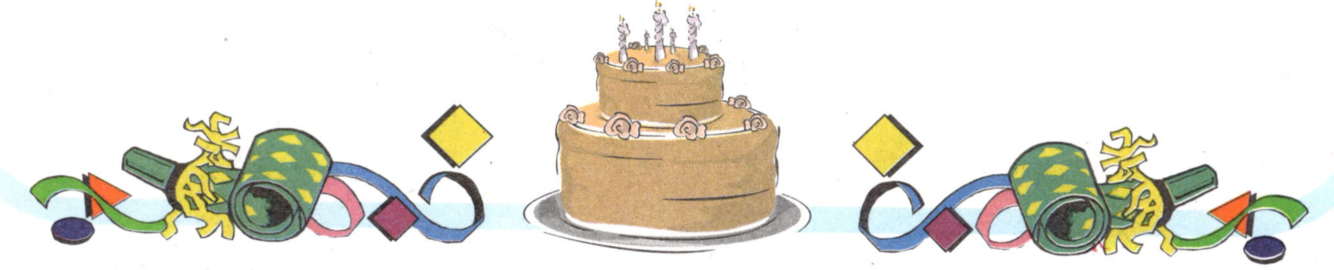

MORE PHOTOGRAPHS

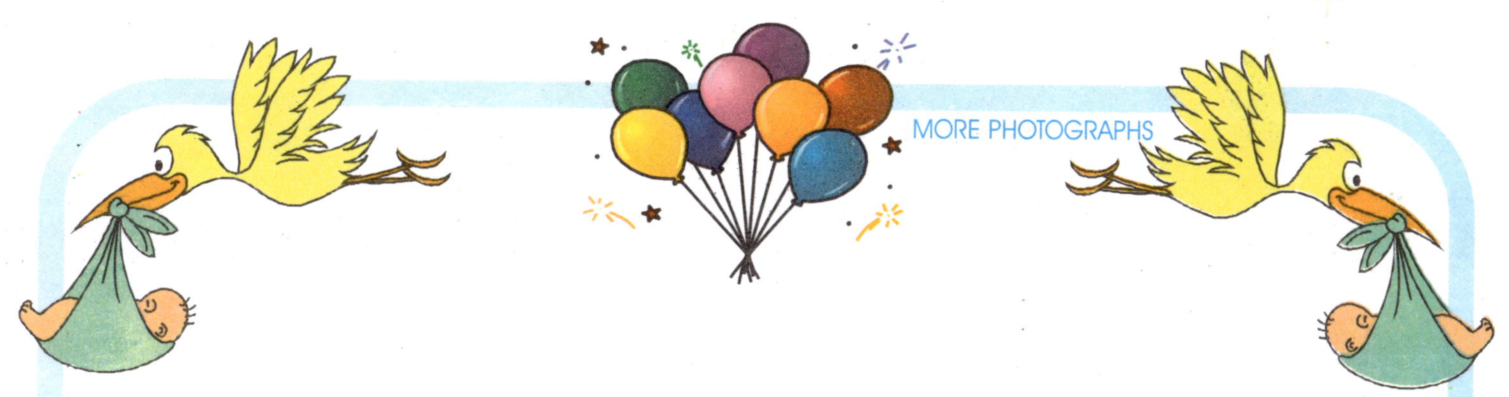

MORE PHOTOGRAPHS

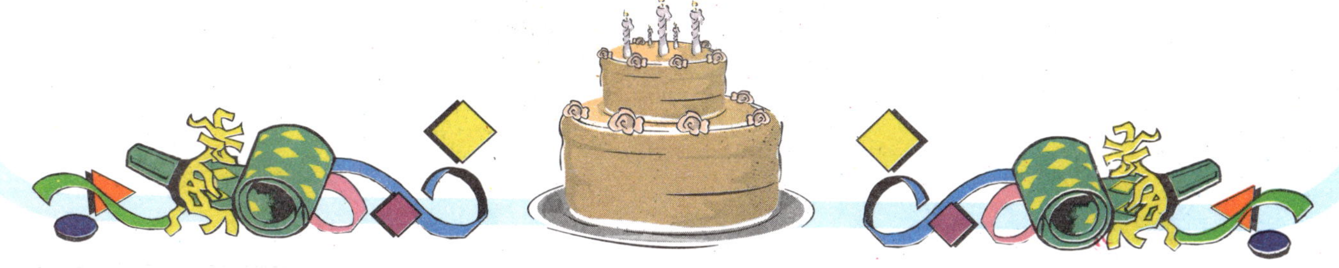

MORE PHOTOGRAPHS

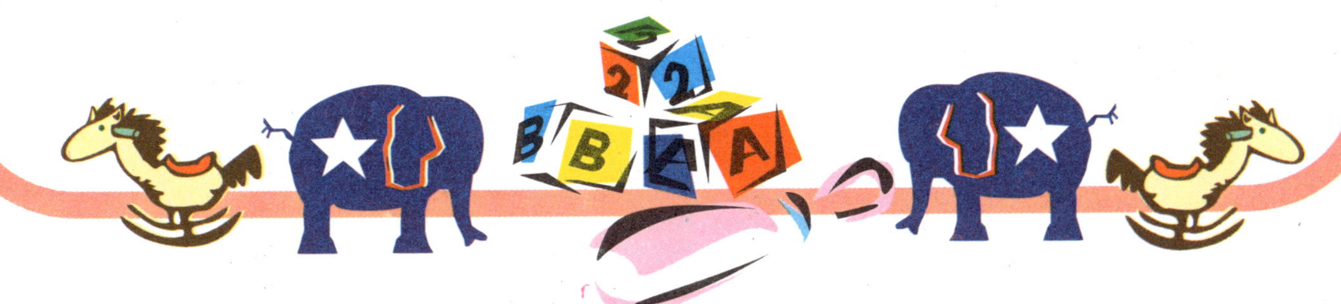

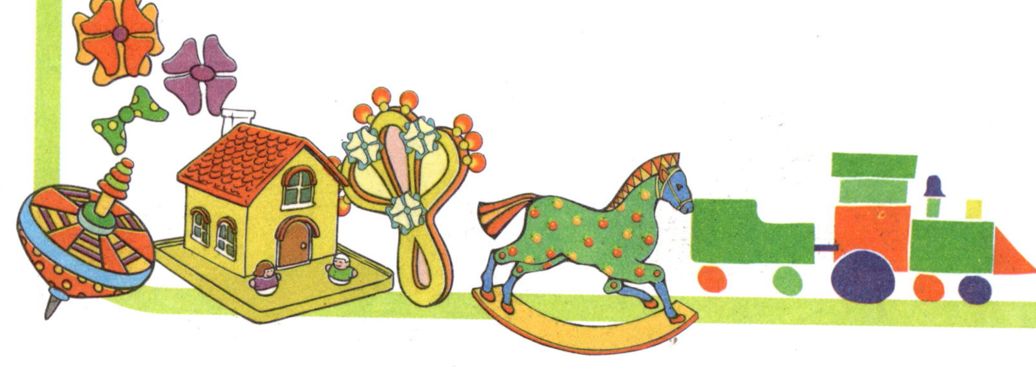

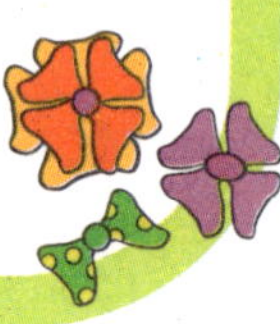

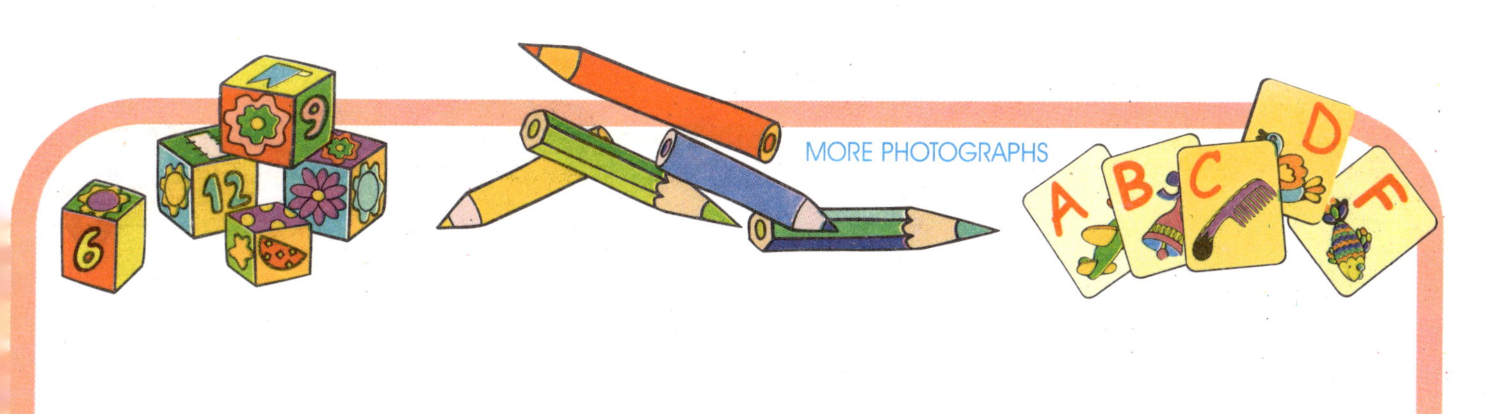
MORE PHOTOGRAPHS

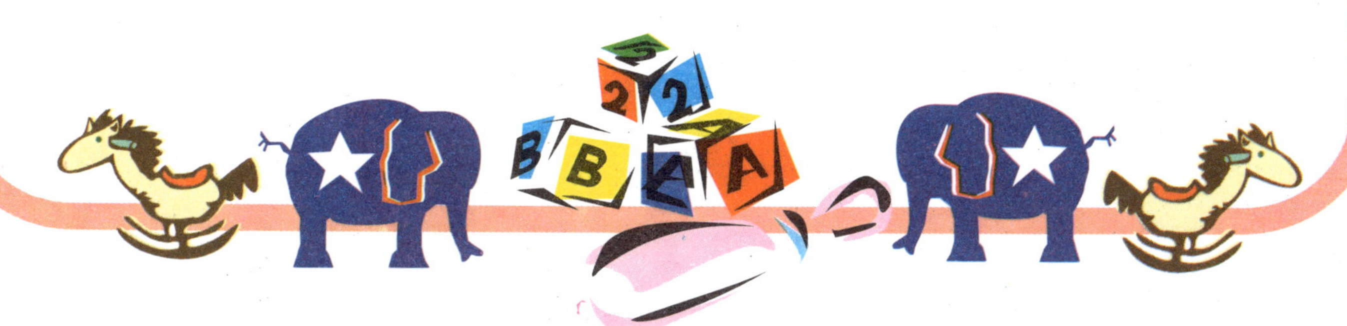

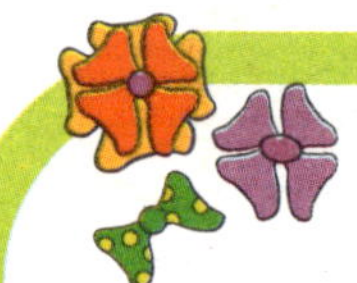

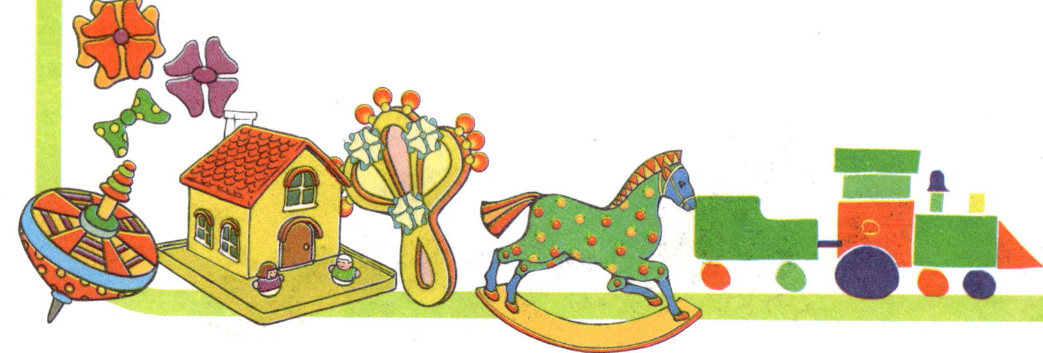

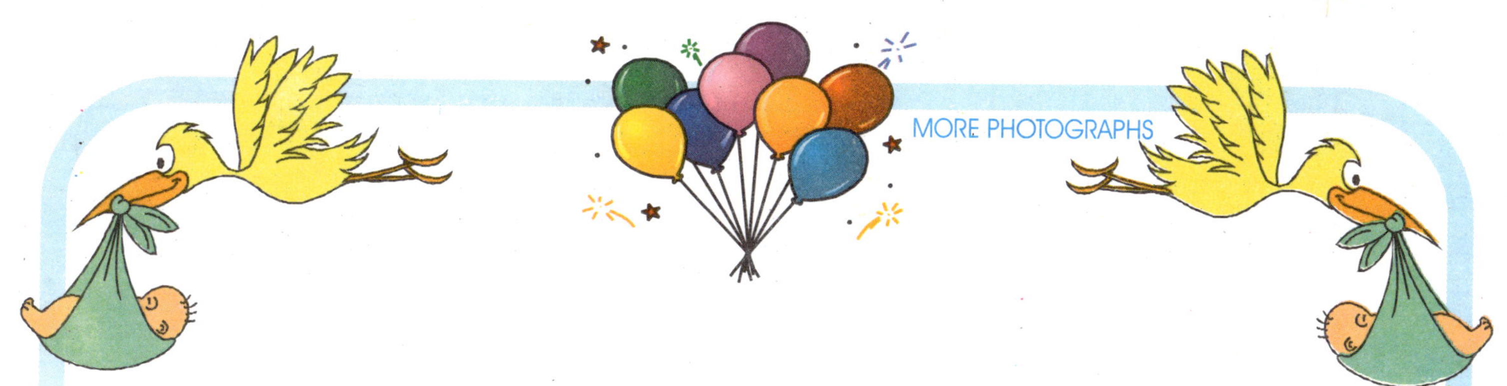
MORE PHOTOGRAPHS

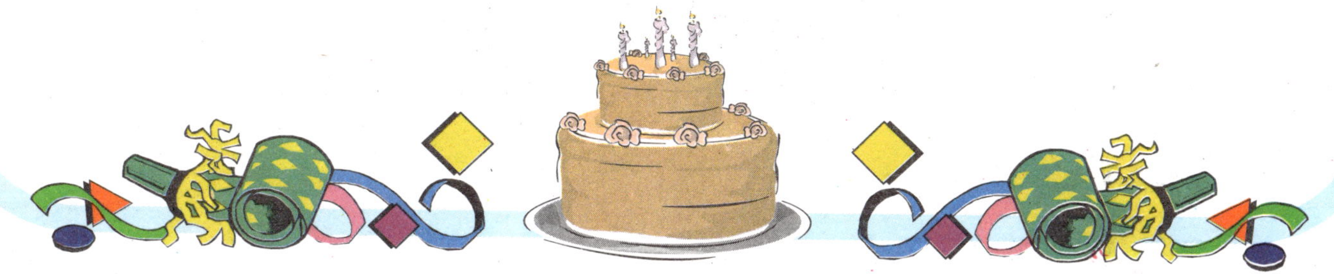

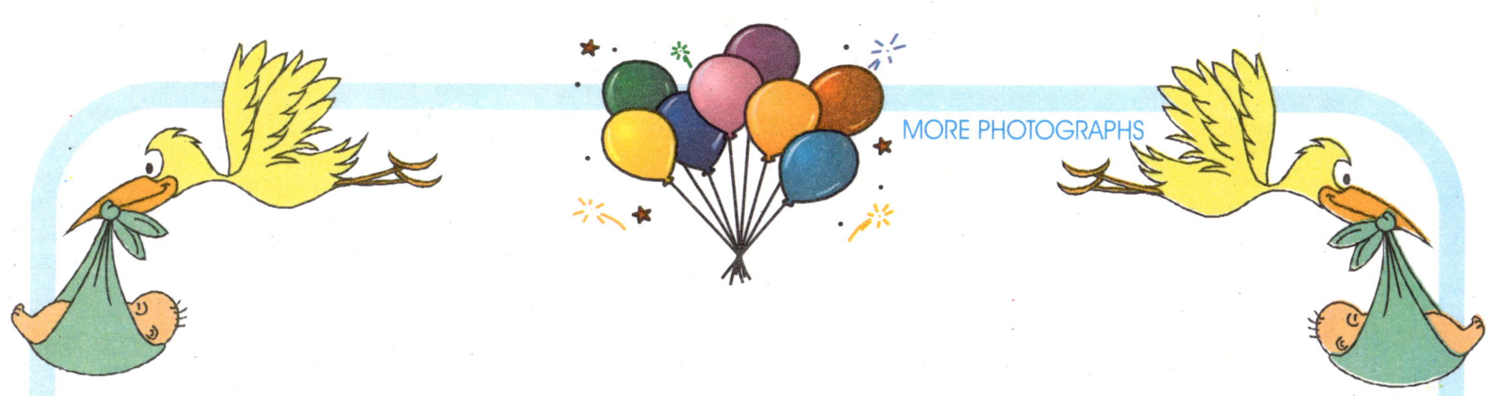
MORE PHOTOGRAPHS

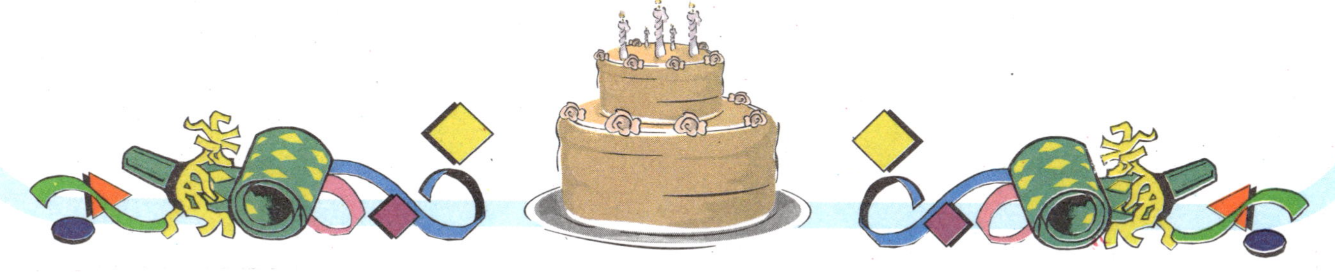

MORE PHOTOGRAPHS

MORE PHOTOGRAPHS

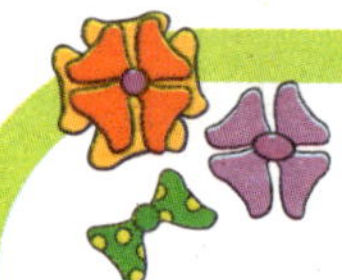

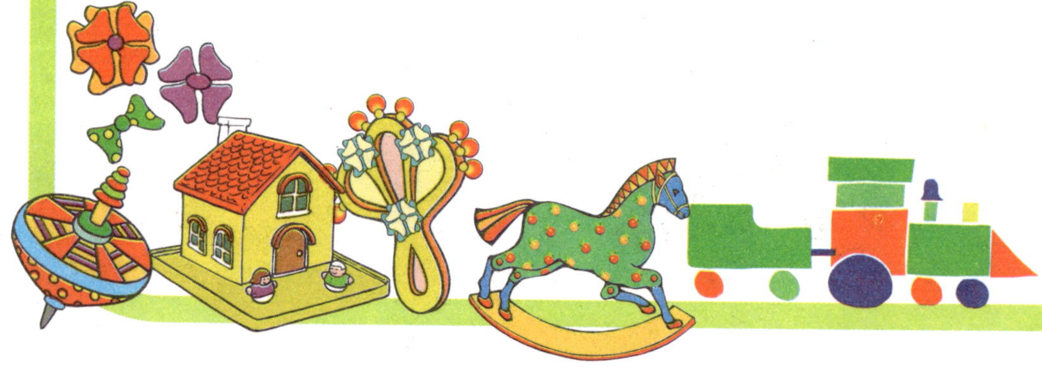

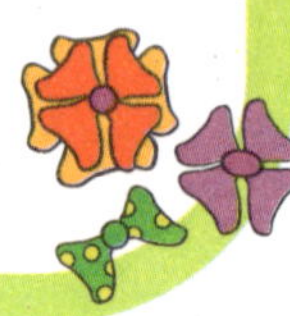

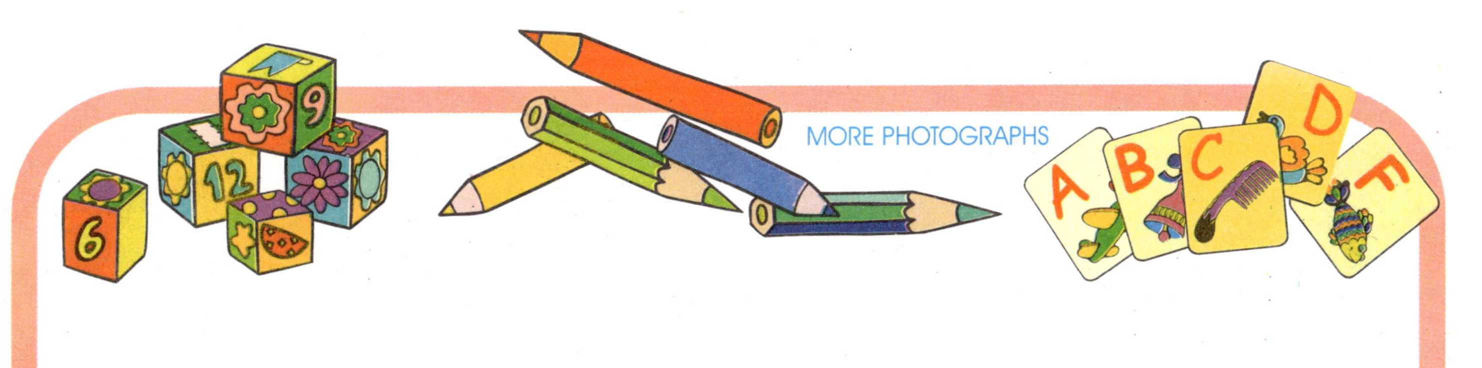

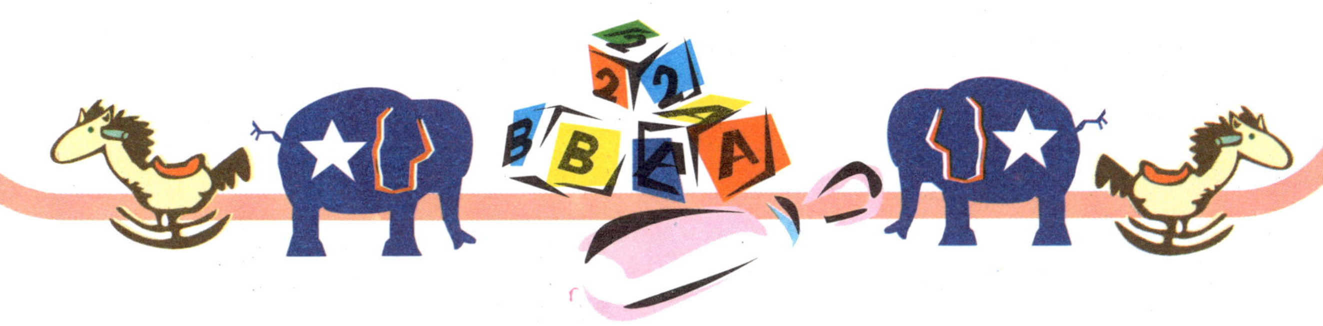

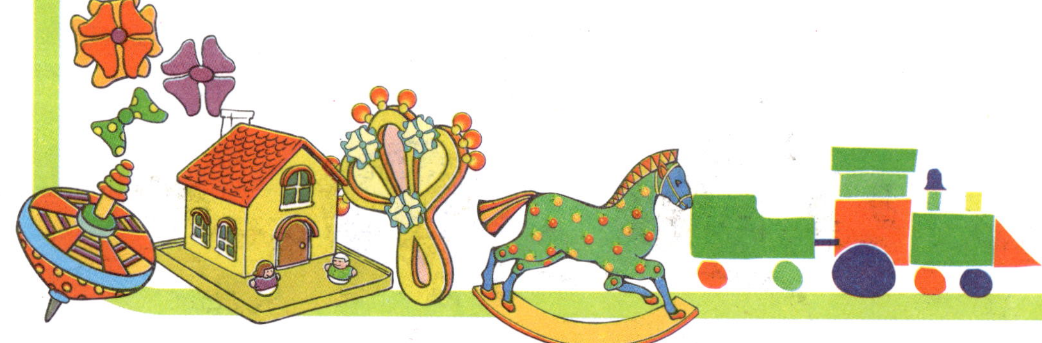

Average Height and Weight of Indian Children

Age	Height (in cms)		Weight (in kgs)	
	Boys	Girls	Boys	Girls
Birth time	49.2-39.3	49.8-39.0	3.1-2.4	2.9-2.4
3 Months	60.1-48.1	59.2-47.4	5.7-4.6	5.5-4.4
6 Months	66.3-53.1	64.5-51.6	7.5-6.0	6.9-5.5
9 Months	70.5-56.4	68.5-54.8	8.7-7.0	7.9-6.3
1 Year	73.4-58.8	72.1-57.7	9.5-7.6	8.7-7.0
1 ½ Years	79.3-63.4	77.7-62.2	10.7-8.6	9.6-7.7
2 Years	84.5-67.6	82.1-65.7	11.7-9.3	10.6-8.5
2 ½ Years	88.9-71.2	86.5-69.2	12.9-10.4	11.8-9.4
3 Years	92.7-74.1	90.0-72.0	13.6-10.9	12.6-10.1
3 ½ Years	95.8-76.7	94.6-75.7	14.5-11.6	13.2-11.0
4 Years	98.1-78.5	98.0-78.4	14.9-11.9	14.3-11.4
4 ½ Years	103.2-82.4	101.1-80.8	16.0-12.8	15.1-12.1
5 Years	106.7-85.4	104.4-83.5	17.0-13.6	16.0-12.8
5 ½ Years	110.4-88.3	107.2-85.8	18.0-14.4	16.6-13.3
6 Years	114.6-91.7	109.4-87.5	19.5-15.6	17.2-13.8

Order and Time of Teething of the Child

Teeth	Upper Jaw	Lower Jaw
Central Incisor	7–10 Months	5–7 Months
Lateral Incisor	9–11 Months	10–12 Months
First Molar	12–14 Months	12–16 Months
Canines	16–20 Months	16–20 Months
Second Molar	20–30 Months	20–28 Months

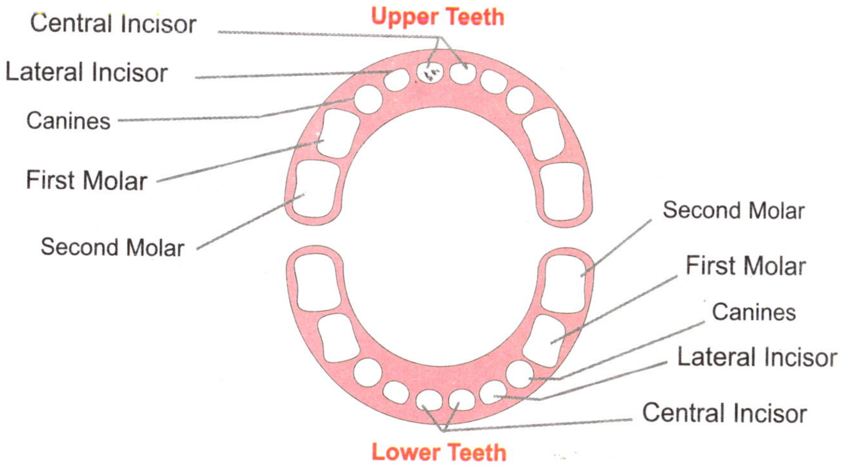

Upper Teeth

Central Incisor

Lateral Incisor

Canines

First Molar

Second Molar

Second Molar

First Molar

Canines

Lateral Incisor

Central Incisor

Lower Teeth

How a Baby Develops in the First Year

Month 1

When a newborn baby is lifted, the head drops. Always support it.

A newborn baby lies with pelvis higher than arms and legs.

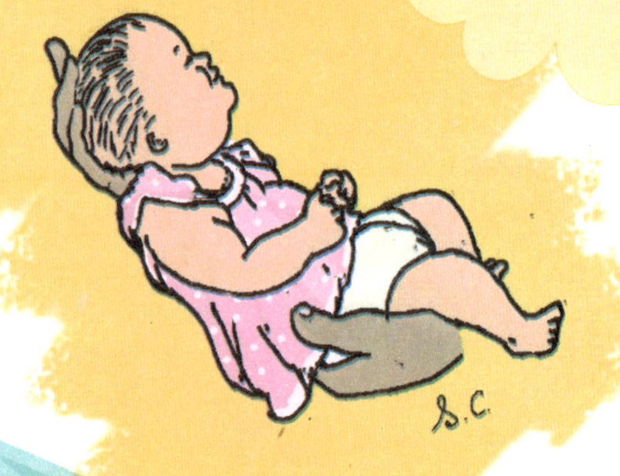

When a newborn baby's palm is touched, the hand closes.

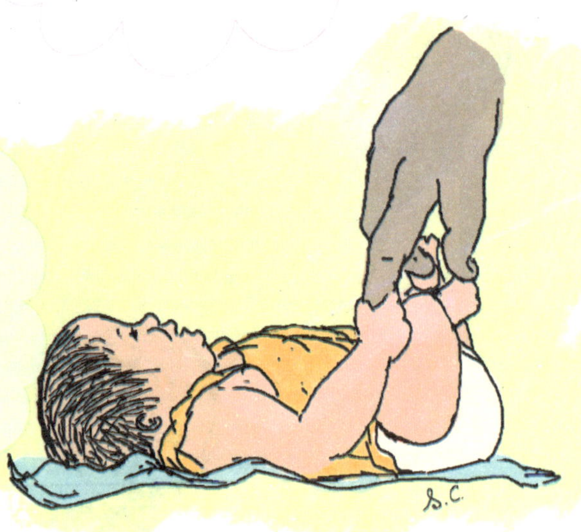

Month 2

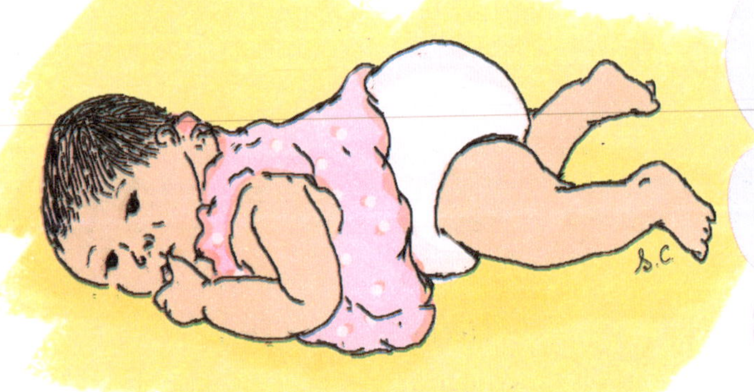

At 2 months, the baby's pelvis is lower and legs are extended.

Month 3

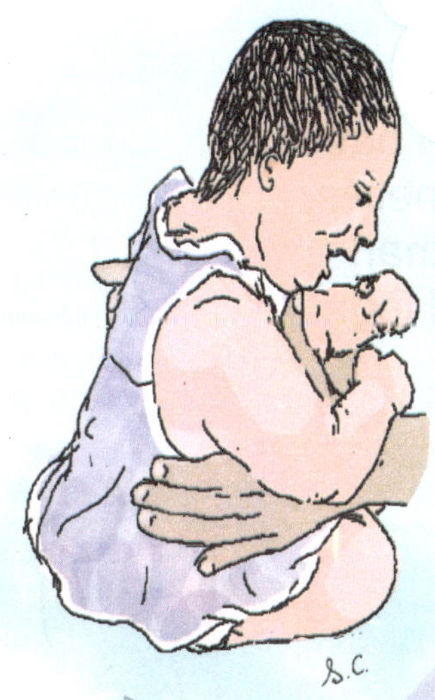

After 2 months, the head is held up when in a sitting position.

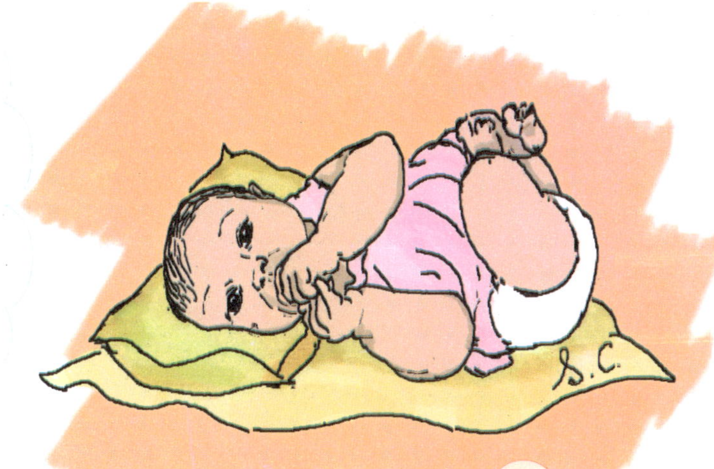

During the 3rd month the baby starts sucking the fist.

Month 4

By 4 months, the baby is able to use the forearms for support.

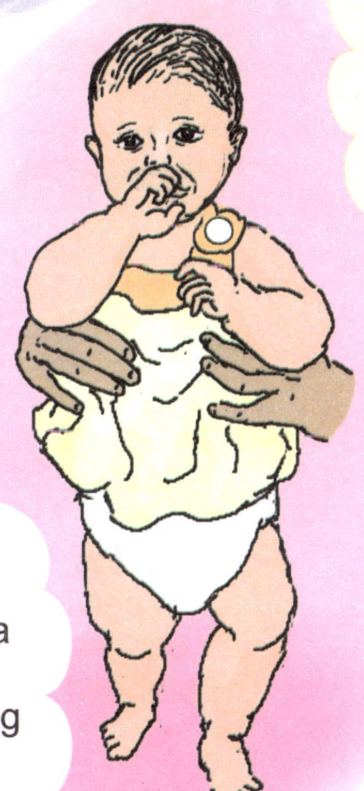

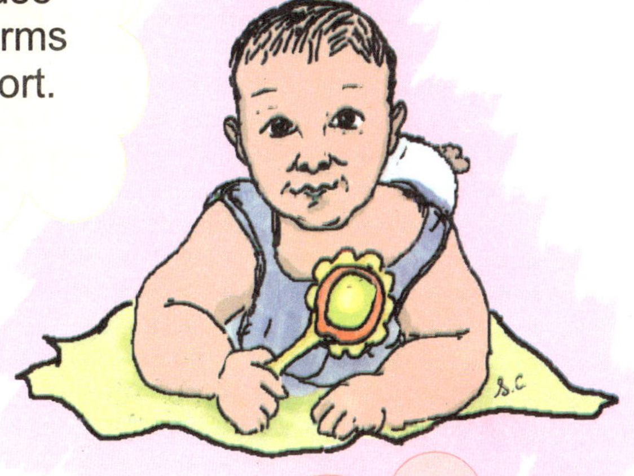

At 4 months, a baby can be held in standing position.

Between 3 and 4 months the baby is able to hold a rattle.

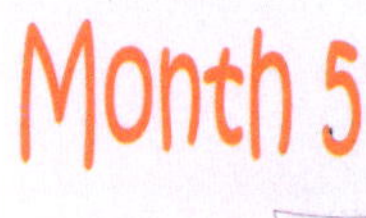

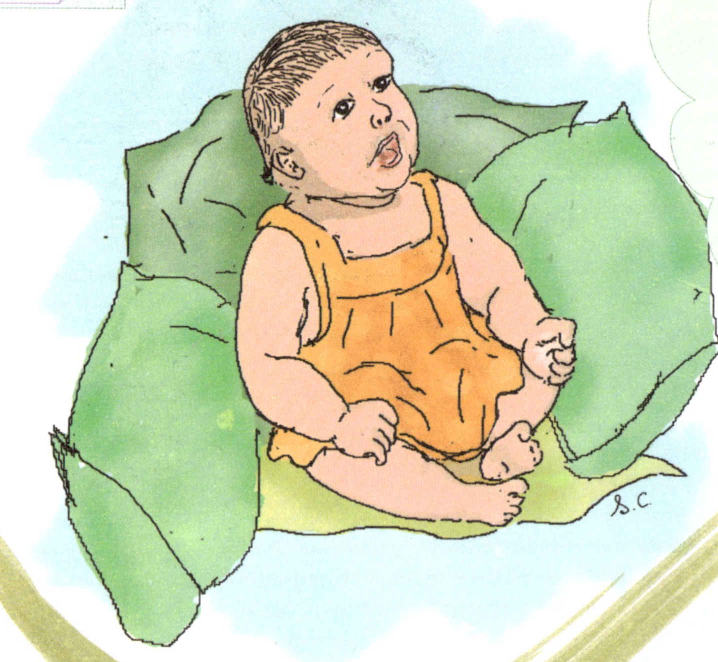

By 5 months the baby can lift chest and head while sitting.

The baby can sit with support, but slips if support is removed.

Month 6

By 6 months, weight is carried on arms which are extended.

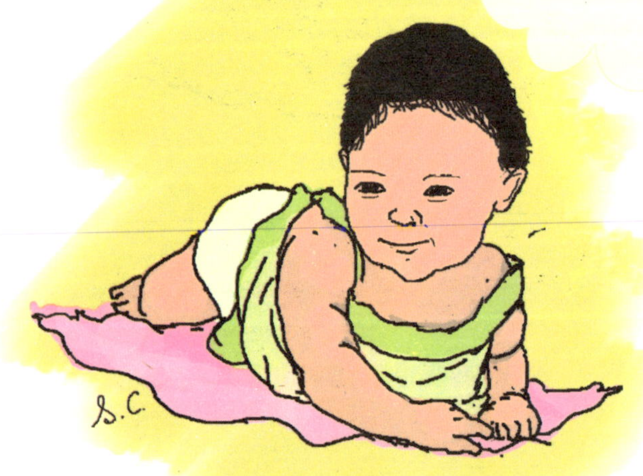

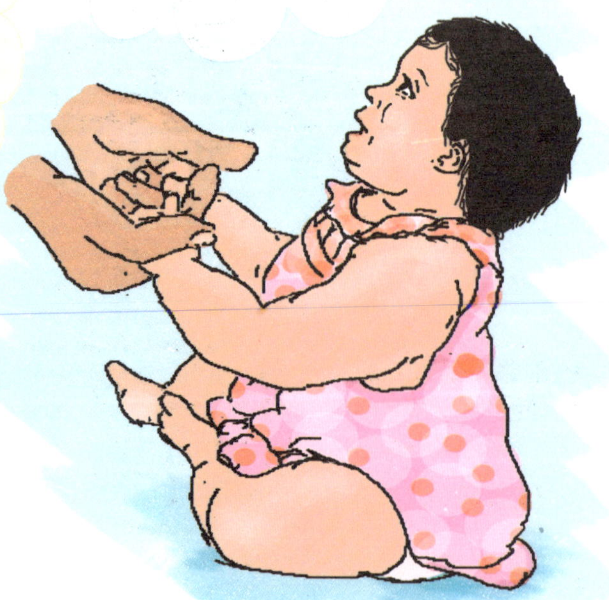

Month 7

By 7 months, the baby uses the hand like a scoop.

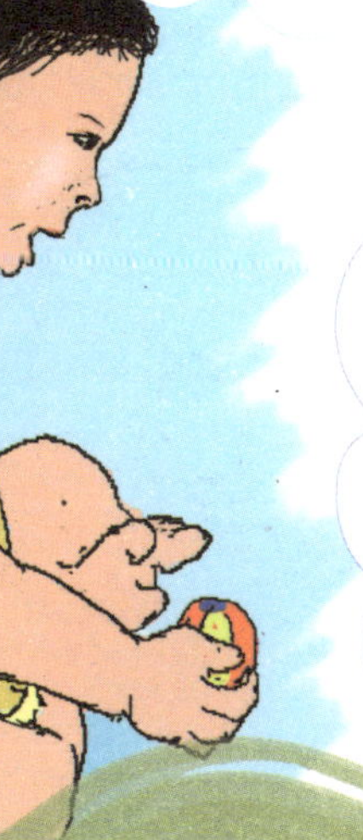

Between 7 & 10 months the baby can sit unsupported.

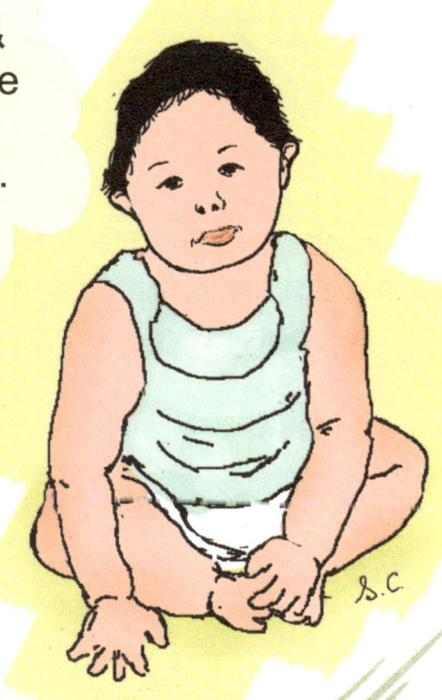

At 7 months, a baby's legs can carry part of its weight if helped.

Month 8

A baby begins sitting up with hand forward for support.

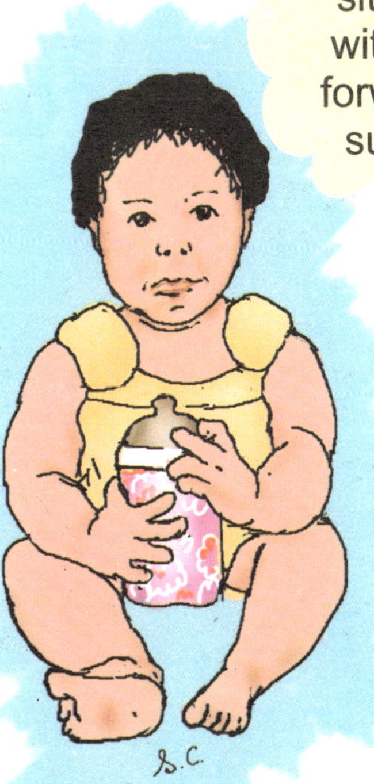

By 8 months, a baby is able to hold a mug in both hands.

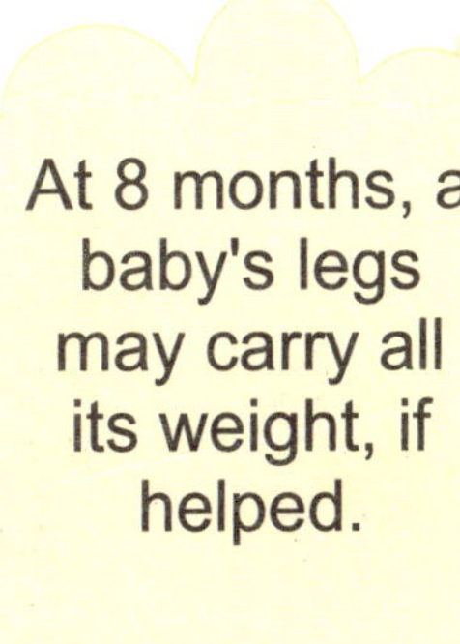

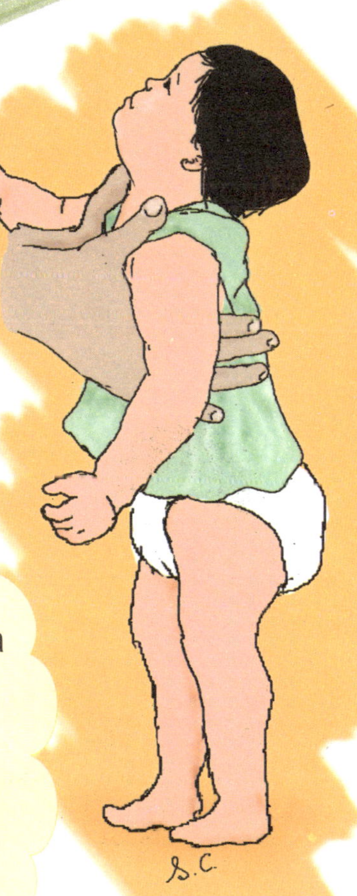

At 8 months, a baby's legs may carry all its weight, if helped.

Month 9

At 9 months, a baby can sit securely for about 10 minutes.

At 9 months, a baby may stand briefly holding onto furniture.

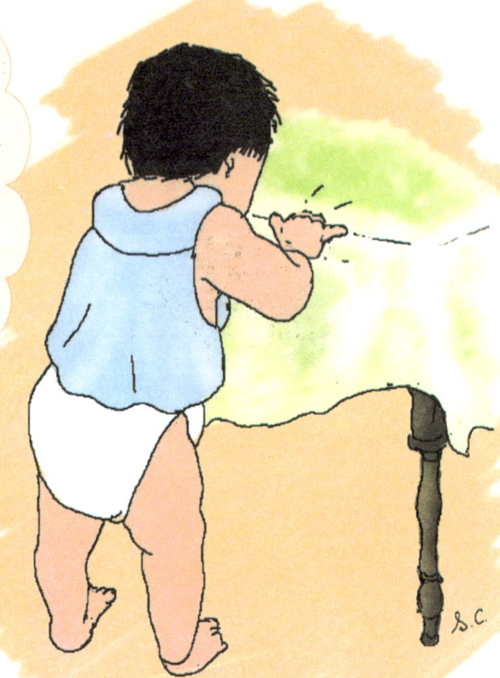

By 9 months, the baby can bring small objects together.

Month 10

At 10 months, a baby learns to clap hands together.

The baby learns to crawl, pulling the body with the hands.

By 10 months, a baby can lean forward to pick up objects.

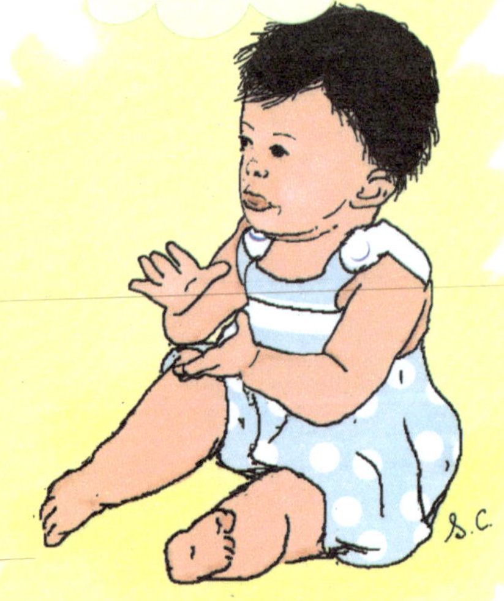

A baby learns to move about a room by holding onto furniture.

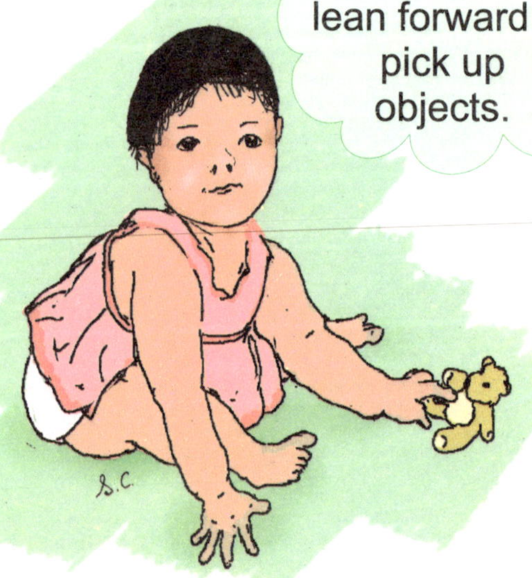

Month 11

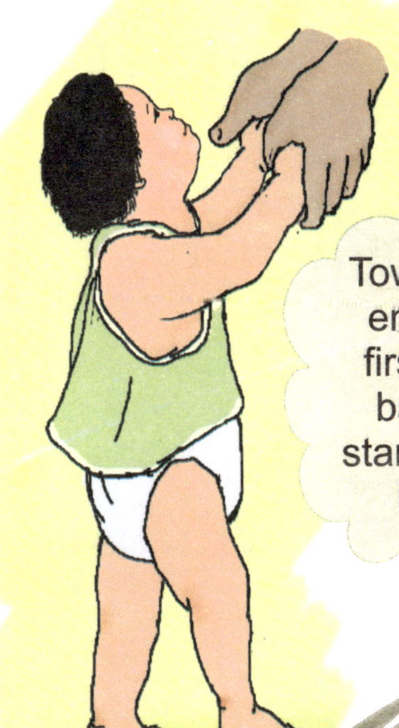

Towards the end of the first year a baby can stand upright if held.

At 11 months, a baby begins to pivot in sitting position.

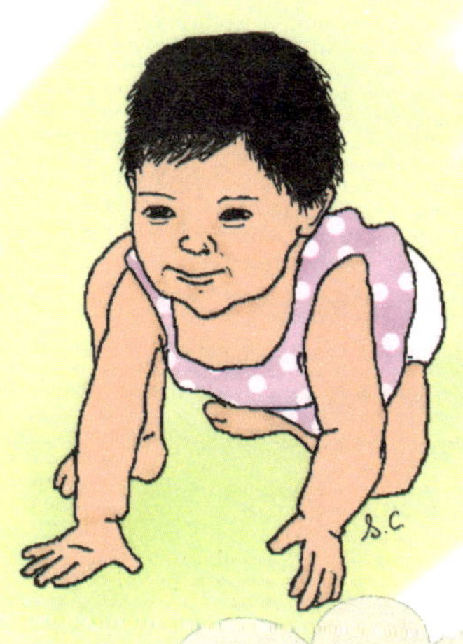

Within another month or so, the baby crawls on hands and knees.

Towards the end of the first year the baby prods with index finger.

Month 12

By one year a baby may be able to move on hands and feet.

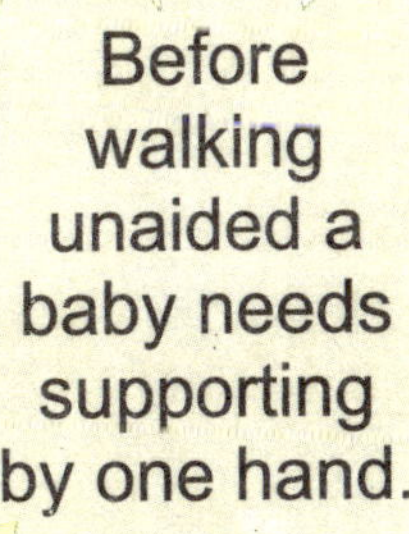

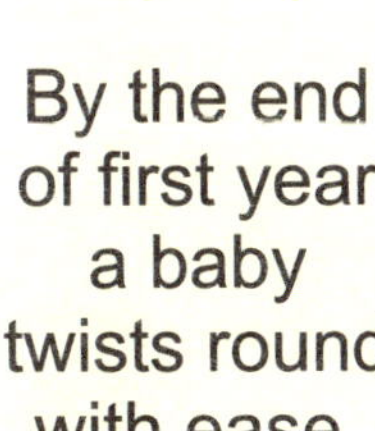

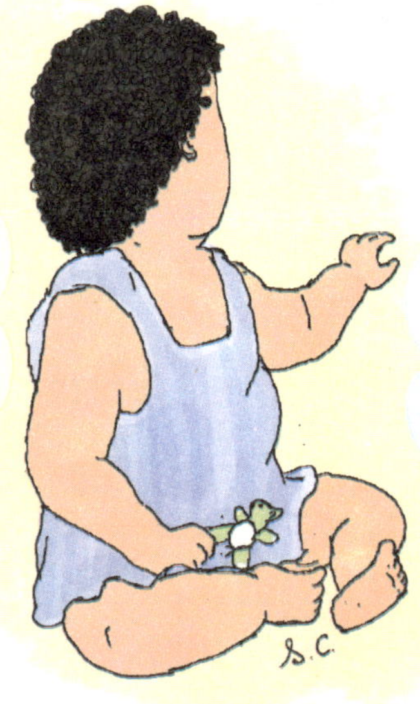

The baby begins picking up with index finger and a thumb.

APPENDIX

VACCINATION TABLE FOR CHILDREN

Disease	Vaccine/Medicine	First Time	Second Time	Third Time
1. Tuberculosis	B.C.G.	At Birth	-	-
2. Whopping Cough, Tetanus and Diphtheria	Triple Antigen D.P.T.	Three times in the first year (6th, 10th & 14th week)	At the age of 1½ years 1st booster	At the age of 5 years 2nd booster
3. Polio	Polio-drops	1st, 6th, 10th & 14 week	1st booster	2nd booster
4. Measles	Vaccine	Between 9 & 12 months	-	-
5. Measles, Mumps, Rubella	M.M.R. Vaccine	15 months	-	-
6. Hepatitis B	Vaccine	At Birth	6 weeks	6-9 months
7. Typhoid	Vaccine	At the age of 3 years	Every 3 years	-
8. Chicken pox	Vaccine	12 months	-	-
9. Meningitis	H.I.B. Vaccine	6th, 10th & 14th week	1½ years 1st booster	-

Points to remember at the time of Vaccination

- ✓Vaccination can be given in minor illnesses like mild fever and cold etc.
- ✓Child suffering from convulsions should not be given diphtheria (Pertusis) vaccine.
- ✓After 4-6 weeks of B.C.G. vaccination, the child develops a small inflamed nodule at the site of vaccination which after sometime subsides on its own.
- ✓After D.P.T. vaccination, the child usually develops mild fever within 24 hours which subsides in one or two days.
- ✓After 2-4 days of measles of M.M.R. vaccination, the child may develop mild fever and rash which subside on their own.

The ratio of increase in height and weight during first five years

Age	Weight increase (per week)
0—3 months	200 grams
4—6 months	150 grams
7—9 months	100 grams
9—12 months	75—50 grams
	Weight increase (per week)
1—2 years	2.5 kilograms
3—5 years	2.0 kilograms

Age	Height increase (per week)
First year	25 cms
Second year	12 cms
Third year	9 cms
Fourth year	7 cms
Fifth year	6 cms